THE

DOMESTIC PHYSICIAN,

AND

FAMILY ASSISTANT,

IN FOUR PARTS:

PART I.—A short System of Anatomy.
II.—On Materia Medica, or a Description of Medicinal Vegetables.
III.—On Pharmacy, or the preparation of Medicines.
IV.—On Physiology, or the description and treatment of Diseases.

BY MARLIN GARDNER & BENJAMIN H. AYLWORTH,
BOTANIC PHYSICIANS.

APPLEWOOD BOOKS
Bedford, Massachusetts

The Domestic Physician and Family Assistant was originally published by H. and E. Phinney of Cooperstown, N.Y. in 1836. The background print on the cover of this edition is taken from the embossing on the original 1836 edition.

Thank you for purchasing an Applewood Book. Applewood reprints America's lively classics—books from the past that are still of interest to modern readers. For a free copy of our current catalog, write to: Applewood Books, P.O. Box 365, Bedford, MA 01730

ISBN 1-55709-583-3

Library of Congress Control Number: 2001095340

PREFACE.

THE preparation of the following pages for the press, has been a work of no small labor and difficulty; for it must appear evident, that to select and condense, on systematic principles, the matter for a work of this character, would require no inconsiderable research and application. Yet the authors feel confident that the public will find, in the "*Family Physician*," a work of equal, if not superior claims, on the score of practical utility, to those of any similar undertaking of the present day. There are several reasons which have induced the authors to publish this work. Notwithstanding much has been done in the way of medical reform, by the establishment of medical schools and colleges on botanic principles, and that numerous students have graduated in these colleges, yet popular prejudice is not sufficiently removed to allow these graduates a fair opportunity for practising in every part of the country—consequently many families are deprived of the attendance of a Botanic Physician. In some parts of the country, interested and designing men have, through their influence, procured the passage of laws which prohibit the Botanic practitioner from receiving compensation for his services, unless he shall first have spent some years in studying the nature and use of *mineral poisons*, how well soever he might otherwise be informed.

Numerous botanic medical works have been published; but they are either quite deficient, or such exhorbitant prices are required for them, that many are disposed to consider them as an imposition, and others do not feel able to buy them. Many are consequently reduced to the sad alternative, when seized with disease, of taking medicines which, although they may remove the present disease, perhaps destroy or debilitate the constitution, and engender worse diseases than are cured—whereas, the vegetable medicines described in this work, remove all curable diseases with the utmost facility, and without the least danger of producing any deleterious effects. This work may appear deficient in some points; but as it is designed for a family assistant, and consequently exposed to the inspection of all classes, the authors think it may be most expedient to supply this deficiency by another work, on the diseases of women and children and practical obstetrics. Sufficient directions are however given, for any common case.

It has been the object of the authors in this work, to render it as brief and intelligible as possible, hoping that the public will cast over its imperfections the gentle mantle of charity—not that we are in the least disposed, however, to beg a truce with critics.

PART I.

A SHORT SYSTEM OF ANATOMY.

OF THE STRUCTURE OF BONES.

THE human bones, in their natural state, are of a dull, white colour. Their texture is varied, not only in different parts of the skeleton, but in different parts of the same bone. Thus in long bones the middle portion is compact, with a cavity in the centre ; the extremities are cellular, or spongy, and the central cavities are occupied by a net work formed of thin plates and fibres.

In a sound state bones have no sensibility, but pain is often felt in them when diseased.

Modern chemistry has ascertained that the earthy matter of bones is principally a phosphate of lime ; carbonate of lime is also found in smaller quantity in them. These earthy substances compose nearly one half the weight of bones ; and a large proportion of the remainder appears to be gelatinous and cartilaginous matter. Bones are supplied with blood vessels, absorbent vessels, and nerves, which enter them by small sinuses, or holes, from which they receive nutrition or support.

The bones are also invested or covered with a membrane denominated periosteum, which is of a fibrous texture. The external surface of the periosteum is connected with the contiguous parts by cellular membrane ; the internal surface is connected with the bone by a great number of fibres, and of blood vessels ; the orifices of these vessels appear when the periosteum is separated from the bone.

OF CARITLAGES, AND THEIR STRUCTURE.

Cartilages are white elastic substances, much softer than bones, in consequence of a much smaller quantity of earth entering into their composition. They have no concelli, or internal membranes, for lodging marrow, nor do they possess any sensibility in a sound state.

One set of cartilages supplies the place of bone, and by their flexibility admit of a certain degree of motion, while their elasticity enables them to recover their natural position, as in the nose, larynx, cartilages of the ribs, &c.

Another set in children supplies the place of bone, until bone can be formed and afford a nidus for the osseus fibres to shoot in, as in the long bones of children.

A third set, and that the most extensive, by the smoothness and lubrication of their surface, allow the bones to move readily, without any abrasion,as in the cartilage of the joints.

A fourth set supplies the office both of cartilage and ligaments, giving the elasticity of the former and flexibility of the latter, as in the bones of the spine and pelvis.

OF THE FORMATION OF BONE.

The generality of bones, and particularly those that are long, are originally formed in cartilage; some, as those of the skull, are formed between membranes; and the teeth, in distinct bags. When ossification is about to commence in any particular part of a cartilage, most frequently in the centre, the arteries which were formerly transparent become dilated, and receive the red blood, from which the osseous matter is secreted. This matter retains for some time the form of the vessel that gives it origin, till more arteries being by degrees dilated, and more osseous matter deposited, the bone at length attains its complete form. During the progress of ossification the surrounding cartilage by degrees disappears, not by being changed into bone, but by an absorption of its parts, the newly formed bone occupying its place.

Some bones are completely formed at the time of birth, as the small bones of the ear. The generality of bones are incomplete until the age of puberty, or between the fifteenth and twentieth year.

Of the Terms used in the Description of Bones, and their Articulations.

The study of Anatomy has been rendered more difficult by the unnecessary introduction of many hard words and arbitrary terms; but some of them are so generally used in the popular works of the present day, that they ought to be understood, and cannot well be dispensed with until a general system of anatomy shall be published in a more simple style.

The word *process* signifies any protuberance or eminence arising from a bone.

Particular processes receive their names from their supposed resemblance to certain objects, and their names are very often composed of two Greek words. Thus the term *caracoid*, which is applied to a well known process, is derived from two Greek words, which signify *crow* and *resemblance*. If a process has a spherical form, it is called a *head*. If the head is flattened on the sides, it is denominated a *condyle*.

A rough protuberance is called a *tuberosity*. A ridge on the surface of a bone is called a *spine*.

The term *apophysis* is nearly synonymous with process; it signifies a protuberance that has grown out of the bone, and is used in opposition to the term *epiphysis*, which signifies a portion of bone growing up on another, but distinct and separable from it, as is the case in infancy with the extremities of the long bones.

Symphysis does not merely imply the connection of bones originally separated, as its derivation imports, but it is understood also to mean the connection of bones by intermediate substances.

Of the skeleton, and its different parts—and the individual bones of which they are composed.

The bones of an animal, arranged and connected with each other in their natural order, separate from the soft parts, compose a skeleton. The skeleton is said to be natural when the bones are connected by their own ligaments, which have been allowed to remain for that purpose. It is called artificial when the bones are connected by wire, or any foreign substance. The artificial skeleton is best calculated for the study of the motions of the different bones, because the dry and hard ligaments of the natural skeleton do not allow the bones to move. The skeleton is divided into the head, the trunk, the superior and inferior extremities.

OF THE HEAD.

The head comprehends the skull, or cranium, and face. The cranium consists of eight distinct bones, which when placed in their natural order form a large spheroidal cavity, for containing the brain, with many foramina, or apertures, that communicate with it. These bones are of a flattened form; they are composed of two tables or plates, with a cellular structure or open net work between them, called *meditullium*, or *deplio*; also some blood vessels. The periosteum, which is on their external surface, is called *pericranium*. Internally, the *dura mater*, or membrane which covers the brain, supplies the place of periosteum.

There are eight of these bones, which are thus denominated—*os frontis*, *ossa paritalia*, *ossa temporum*, *os occipitis*, *os sphenoids*, and *os ethmoides*. The os frontis, as its name imports, forms the front part of the cranium, (or the forhead,) and the upper portion of the orbits of the eyes. The two ossa paritalia form the upper and middle portion, between the os frontis, and vertere, or crown of the head. The two ossa temporum compose the lower part of the sides of the head above and around the ears. The os occipitis makes the whole hinder part, and some of the base. The os ethmoides is placed between the orbits of the eyes. The os sphenoides extends across the base of the cranium, and is in contact with most of the other bones of the cranium, and some of those of the face, and supports the brain which rests on it.

SUTURES.

The above mentioned bones are joined to each other by five sutures, (or a kind of seems,) the names of which are—the *coronal*, *lambdoidal*, *sagittal*, and two *squamose*.

The coronal suture is extended over the head, from or

within about an inch of one of the eyes, to the like ais-tance from the other.

The lambdoidal suture begins some way below, and farther back than the vertex, or crown of the head, whence its two legs ar stretched downwards, and to each side of the head some way back of the ears.

The sagittal suture is placed longitudinally in the middle of the upper part of the skull, and commonly terminates at the middle of the coronal and lambdoidal sutures, between which it is placed as an arrow between the bow and string. This suture is sometimes continued through the middle of the os frontis down to the root of the nose.

The squamose agglutinations, or false sutures, are on each side of the head, a little above the ear, of a semicircular figure, formed by the overlapping, (like one scale upon another) of the upper part of the temporal bones, on the lower part of the parietal, where in both bones there are a great many small risings and furrows.

OF THE FACE.

The face is an irregular pile of bones, composing the front and under part of the head, and is divided into the upper and lower maxilla, or jaws.

The upper jaw consists of six bones on each side, of one single bone placed in the middle, and of sixte n teeth. The thirteen bones are, two *ossa maralaria superiora*, two *ossa nasi*, two *ossa unguis*, two *ossa malarum*, two *ossa palati*, two *ossa spongiosa inferiora*, and the *vomer*. The ossa maralaria superiora form the principal part of the cavity of the nose, with the whole lower and fore part of the upper jaw, and a large proportion of the roof of the mouth. The ossa nasi are placed at the upper and front part of the nose. The ossa unguis are at the internal angles of the orbits of the eyes. The ossa palati in the back part of the palate, extending upward to the orbits of the eyes. The ossa spongiosa in the lower part of the cavity of the nose ; and the vomer is the partition whichseparates the two nostrils.

THE TEETII.

The teeth in an adult, when they are perfect, are sixteen

in each jaw. They are four kinds, viz.—*incisores*, *cuspidati*, *bicuspides*, and *molares*. On each side, supposing it divided in the middle, there are two incisores, one cuspidatus, two bicuspides, and three molares. The incisores are the front teeth.

OF THE TRUNK.

The trunk consists of the spine, thorax, and pelvis.

THE SPINE.

The spine is the long pile of bones extending from the conduits of the occipit to the end of the os coccyigis (called the back bone.) The spine is not straight, its upper part being drawn backward by strong muscles; it gradually advances forward to support the osophagus vessels of the head, &c. Then it turns backward to make room for the heart and lungs. It is next bent forward, to support the viscera of the abdomen. It afterwords turns backward for the enlargement of the pelvis; and lastly it is reflected forward for supporting the lowest great intestines.

THE VERTEBRÆ.

The vertebræ are divided into the true and false. The true vertebræ are the twenty-four upper bones of the spine, on which the several motions of the trunk of the body are performed. The true vertebræ are divided into three classes, which agree wit[illegible] other in their general structure, but are distinguish[illegible]y several peculiarities. These classes are named *cervical*, *dorsal*, and *lumbar*.

The cervical are the seven uppermost; the twelve next below are the dorsal; and the five next below are called lumbar vertebræ, (and form that portion of the spine called the small of the back.)

FALSE VERTEBRÆ.

The lower pyramid, or under part of the spine, consists of one large triangular bone, called the os sacrum, and some smaller bones denominated the os coccygis.

THE THORAX.

The thorax resembles a flattened cone, cut away obliquely at its basis, and regularly truncated at its apex.

It is formed by the dorsal vertebræ behind the ribs on the sides, and the sternum (or breast bone) before.

THE RIBS

Are long crooked bones, placed in an oblique direction downwards as respects the spine. Their number is generally twelve, but eleven or thirteen on each side have been found. The ribs are commonly divided into true and false. The true ribs are the seven uppermost on each side. Their cartilages are all gradually longer as they descend and are joined to the breast bone. They inclose the heart and lungs. The five inferior ribs of each side are the false ribs, whose cartilages do not reach the sternum. To these ribs the circular edges of the diaphragm (or midriff) is connected.

THE STERNUM

Is the broad flat bone in the front part of the thorax, called the breast bone. In adults it is composed of three pieces which appear after the cartilages connecting them are destroyed. The ribs are articulated to the spine behind and to the sternum before, in a way which admits of a compound motion.

THE PELVIS.

The pelvis is the cavity at the lower part of the trunk, formed by the os sacrum and os coccygis, (the lower divisions of the back bone) and the ossa innominenta, or what are called the hip bones. The ossa innominenta are one on each side, and are connected with the sacrum behind, and to each other, by the intervention of a cartilage in front. They form, with the back bone, the whole of the bones which encircle the lower part of the trunk of the body. The two points of bone on which we rest when in a sitting posture, are processes, or a continuation of ossa innominenta. The acetabulum, or socket for receiving the head of the os femoris, or thigh bone, is about the middle of each ossa innominenta, on the outside.

OF THE SUPERIOR EXTREMITIES.

The superior extremities include the shoulder, the arm,

the fore-arm, and the hand. The shoulder is composed of the clavicle and scapula. The clavicle (or collar-bone) is a long crooked bone, which is placed horizontally between the sternum and upper front part of the scapula, (or shoulder blade.)

THE SCAPULA,

Or shoulder blade, is the triangular bone situated on the back and upper part of the thorax. The use of the scapula is to serve as a fulcrum to the arm, and by altering its position on different occasions, a socket to move in, always properly situated, (which is called the glenoid cavity) and thereby to assist and enlarge the motions of the arm and shoulder.

THE ARM.

The arm is that portion between the elbow and shoulder, and has but one bone, which is best known by the Latin name of the *os humeri*; it is long, round, and nearly straight. The upper end consists of a round, smooth head, which is articulated with the glenoid cavity by the capsular ligament, to form the shoulder joint.

THE FORE-ARM

Is that portion of the arm between the elbow and wrist, and consists of two bones, one of which is called radius, from its supposed resemblance to the spoke of a wheel, and the other ulna, from its being used as a measure. These bones are concerned in very different operations. The ulna forms the elbow joint with the os humeri; the radius is the moveable basis of the hand. When the palm of the hand is held toward the face, with the thumb outward, these two bones will be parallel, the radius on the outside, and the ulna inside.

THE HAND.

The hand comprehends the whole structure from the end of the radius, (or bones of the fore-arm) to the points of the fingers, including the thumb.

The hand consists of the *carpus*, or wrist, the *metacarpus*, or palm of the hand, and the fingers, among which the thumb is reckoned.

THE CARPUS.

The carpus, (or wrist) is composed of eight small bones, arranged in two rows, one of which rows is attached to the bones of the fore-arm, and the other to the body of the hand. They are arranged in the following order, beginning with the external bone of the first row, to wit: *os scaphoides*, *lunare*, *cuneiforme*, *pisiform*, *trapezium*, *trapezoids*, *magnum*, and *unciform*.

THE METACARPUS

Consists of four bones, which compose the body, or palm of the hand, and sustain the fingers.

THE THUMB AND FINGERS.

The thumb and four fingers are each composed of three bones. The regular arrangement of the bones of the fingers has obtained for them the name of the three *phalanges*. The bones of each finger bear a strong resemblance to those of the others, in every particular.

THE INFERIOR EXTREMITIES.

The inferior extremities consist of the thigh, leg and foot.

THE THIGH

Consists of one bone only, the *os femoris*, which is very strong, and larger than any other bone of the skeleton. It is nearly cylindrical in the middle, and slightly curved. The upper extremity is a spherical head, connected with the body of the bone by a neck which stands obliquely outward, which causes the bodies of the bones to stand farther apart than the heads where they enter the acetabulum, or sockets.

THE LEG

Is composed of two bones, the *tibia* and *fibula*. The *patella*, (or knee-pan,) being evidently appropriated to the knee joint, may be regarded as common to both the thigh and leg.

THE TIBIA

Is the long, thick, triangular bone, situated in the internal part of the leg, and continued in almost a straight line with the thigh bone, and is commonly called the *shin bone.*

THE FIBULA

Is the small bone placed on the outside of the leg, opposite the external angle of the tibia—the shape of it is irregular.

THE PATELLA

Is the small flat bone, situated in the fore part of the knee joint. Its shape resembles the figure of the heart, with its point downwards, and is called the knee pan.

THE FOOT.

The foot is divided into the tarsus, metatarsus, and toes. The side of the great toe is necessarily described as the internal.

TARSUS.

The tarsus consists of seven spongy bones: The *astragalus, os. calcis, naviculare, cuboides, cuniform externum, cuniform medium, cuniform internum.* The os cabeis forms the heel. The astragalus is above the os cabeis, and articulated to it below, and to the tibia and fibula above; and before, to the os naviculare. The os cuniform internum, is placed at the internal side of the tarsus. The cuniform medium stands next; the cuniform externum next; and the os cuboides is at the external or outside of the foot.

METATARSUS.

The metatarsus is composed of five bones, which agree in their general characters with the metacarpal bones of the hand. The metatarsus comprises that part of the foot between the tarsus and toes. The metatarsal bones are distinguished by number, commencing at the internal side.

THE TOES.

The bones of the toes are very similar to those of the thumb and fingers. They are smaller and shorter. The ends are larger in proportion to the middle.

OSTEOLOGY OF MUSCLES IN GENERAL.

That soft, fibrous, red colored substance, which constitutes so large a portion of the volume of animals, is called flesh, or muscle.

By the contraction of this substance, the spontaneous motion of animals is produced; and on that account, the fibres which compose it, have long been regarded with particular attention.

Muscular fibres are not only arranged in those regular masses on the trunk and limbs of the body, which are so familliar to us by the name of muscles, or cords, but they also exist in some of the most important viscera, and produce the internal as well as the external motion of animals.

Muscles, when examined with magnifying glasses, appear to be composed of very fine fibres.

Muscular motion takes place under the following different circumstances:—*First*,—When irritation, or stimulus, is applied directly to the muscular fibre. *Second*,—When irritation is applied to a nerve connected with a muscle. *Third*,—When it is induced by volition. The rapidity with which muscles contract, is surprising, as in the motion of the tongue in rapid speaking. The force of muscular contraction greatly exceeds the power of cohesion. Thus a muscle deprived of life would be completely lacerated by a weight suspended from it, which it could easily raise by its contraction during life. Muscular fibres are situated very differently in different parts.—They compose almost the whole substance of the heart. They also form one of the coats of the stomach and intestines, and of the urinary bladder. Muscles possess great sensibility, and the least puncture or wound excites considerable pain.

It would exceed the proposed limits of this work to enter into even a general description of the muscles. We shall therefore only give a general description of those muscles which are particularly connected with, or concerned in, the various functions of the viscera.

THE DIAPHRAGM.

The diapragm, or midriff, is a broad thin muscle which makes a complete septum or partition between the thorax and abdomen—is concave below, and convex above; the middle of it on each side reaching as high within the thorax as the fourth rib. The fibres of this muscle arise from the internal surface of the thorax, and run like radii from the circumference to the centre of a circle, and are inserted into a cordiform tendon which is situated in the middle of the diaphragm, in which the fibres from opposite sides are interlaced. Toward the right side, the tendon is perforated by a triangular hole, for the passage of the vena cava inferior, (a large blood vessel,) and the upper part of it is connected with the pericardium (or heart-case) and mediastinum. The diaphragm is the principal agent in respiration, particularly in inspiration; for when it is in action, the fibres, from their different attachments, endeavor to bring themselves into a plain toward the middle tendon, by which the cavity of the thorax is enlarged, particularly the sides where the lungs are chiefly situated.

OF THE BRAIN.

The whole of that soft mass which fills the cavity of the cranium is called the Brain. This mass is covered with threo membranes, two of which were called *meninx*, or *maters*, by the ancient anatomists, who believed that all the other membranes of the body originated from them. These membranes are denominated the *dura mater*, *tunica arachnoidea*, and *pia mater*.

The *dua mater* encloses the brain and all its appendages, and lines the different parts of the cranium. This is the thickest and strongest membrane of the body. The dura mater adheres every where to the surface of the cranium, or skull, in the same manner as the periosteum adheres to other bones.

The tunica arachnoidea, is an exceedingly thin, tender, and transparent membrane, in which no vessels have been hitherto observed.

The pia mater, named from its tenderness, is somewhat of the nature of the former covering, but is extremely vascular. It covers the brain in general—enters double between all its convulutions, and lines the different cavities called ventricles.

Of the basis of the Brain, and the Nerves which proceed from it.

When the brain has been carefully detached from the cranium, and the nerves adhering to it are preserved, the olfactory, or first pair of nerves (they are numbered from before backward) appear on the anterior lobes, running nearly parallel to each other, at a small distance from the great fissure. They are flat, and thin and soft in their texture. Their breadth is rather more than one sixth of an inch.

The optic, or second pair of nerves, are smaller than the olfactory, and lead to the eye-balls. The third and to the ninth pairs of nerves arise successively toward the back part of the head, and are distinguished by numbers.

The Medulla Spinalis, or *Spinal Marrow*,

Is continued from the brain through the occipital bone, into the great canal of the spine, and continues to the first lumbar vertebræ. The nerves go off from each side, hence it will be seen that the nerves are all intimately connected with the brain.

Of the Rete Mucosum.

A short description of this substance may be interesting, if not useful. Immediately in contact with the internal surface of the outer coat of the skin, is a very thin structure, of a pulpy or mucilaginous consistence, which appears to be spread uniformly over it, but cannot be detached without deranging its own texture. It can be best examined after the cuticle is raised with a blister. In this pulpy substance resides the pigmentum, or coloring matter, which gives the peculiar complexion to the different races of men. The other two coats of the skin are white, or transparent, but this substance is black in negroes, copper-colored, yellow, or tawny, in many of the Asiatics, and yellow, with a tincture of red, in the aborigines of America, while it is transparent or whitish in Europeans and their descendants.

GLANDS IN GENERAL.

Glands are fleshy, vascular substances, which secrete mucus and other juices, as the saliva, &c. which tend to lubricate and moisten the various parts of the body. But it will exceed the limits of this work to give a minute description of each gland; we shall therefore only give a short preliminary description of the most important.

THE SALIVARY GLANDS.

There are three principal glands on each side of the back part of the mouth; the *parotid*, the *submaxillary*, and the *sublingual*. The salivary fluid secreted by these glands, is inodorous, insipid, and limpid, like water, but much more viscid, and of greater specific gravity. Water constitutes at least four fifths of all its bulk, and animal mucus one half its solid contents. It also contains some albumen, soda, lime, &c. This fluid is supposed to possess a solvent power with respect to food.

The tonsil glands are situated at the entrance of the asophagus, or in what is called the throat. They appear on each side considerably prominent. The epiglottis is situated between the tonsils at the root of the tongue.

OF THE PERICARDIUM.

The pericardium is a membranous sack, that encloses the heart, and keeps that organ in its place by being attached to the diaphragm and blood vessels.

THE HEART.

The heart is composed of muscular fibres, which are so arranged as to give it a conical form, and four distinct cavities within it. Two of these cavities, which are called *auricles*, receive the blood from the veins. The other two cavities communicate with the arteries, and are called ventricles.

The auricles form the lower part of the heart, and the ventricles the middle and upper part. The two great veins called vena cava, which bring the blood from every part of the body, open into the right auricle from above and below. The right auricle opens into the right ventricle ; and from this ventricle arises the artery denominated pulmonary, which passes to the lungs.

The pulmonary veins which bring back the blood from the lungs, open into the left auricle ; this auricle opens into the left ventricle ; and from this ventricle proceeds the *aorta*, or great artery, which carries blood to every part of the body.

These arteries are furnished with valves which are brought into action at each contraction or beat of the heart; hence will be understood the phenomena of pulsation, one of which is produced by every contraction of the heart. Each contraction forces a certain quantity of blood into the arteries, the motion of which may be felt in various parts of the body. There is the same quantity of blood received into the ventricles at each pulsation from the auricles that is thrown from the ventricles into the arteries.

OF THE TRACHEA.

The trachea, or windpipe, commences at the throat, and passes down the neck in front of the osophagus, as low as the third dorsal vertebræ, when it divides into two branches, called bronchia, one of which goes to the right and the other to the left lung.

OF THE LUNGS.

There are two of these organs, each of which occupies one of the cavities of the thorax (or side of the chest.) When placed together in their natural position, they resemble the hoof of an ox, with its back or bottom part forward ; but they are at such distance from each other, and of such figure, as to admit the heart between them.

Each lung is divided, by very deep fissures, into portions called lobes. The right lung is composed of three of these lobes, and the left lung of two.

The lungs are of a soft, spongy texture; they consist of very small cells, which communicate with the trachea, and branches of the trachea that ramify through them in every part.

THE ABDOMEN.

The abdomen comprises the whole space between tne diaphragm above, and os inomminenta, or hip bones.

The abdomen contains the stomach and whole intestinal tube; the liver, the pancreas, and the spleen; the urinary organs, the kidneys, the ureters, and bladder; the peritoneum, the mesentery, and omentum.

THE PERITONEUM.

The peritoneum is a very thin, firm membrane, which is extremely smooth on the internal surface. It lines the whole internal surface of the abdomen, and is reflected and attached to the various viscera in the abdomen.

THE OSOPHAGUS.

The osophagus is a muscular tube which reaches from the mouth, or throat, to the stomach, in which the food passes to the stomach. It is placed between the trachea and spine.

THE STOMACH.

This important organ, which occasionally exerts a powerful influence upon every part of the body, appears very simple in its structure. It is composed of several lamina, or coats, each of a different structure. These coats are:—First, on the outside, a membraneous coat formed by the reflection of the peritoneum; the next coat is called the muscular coat; the third, the nervous coat; the fourth, or internal, is called the villious or velvet coat.

The internal coat of the stomach is covered with a mucus, which is effused upon it by its secreting organs. Besides this mucus, a large quantity of a different fluid, or liquor, the proper gastric juice, or fluid of the stomach, is effused from its surface. This liquor (the gastric) is the principal agent in the process of digestion, or the effect produced by the stomach upon the aliment, or food.

The stomach is situated principally in the left side, immediately below the liver. The upper orifice, or cardia, where the osophagus communicates with the stomach, is nearly opposite the last dorsal vertebrae; and, owing to the curved form of the stomach, the lower orifice, or pylorus, is situated a little to the right of that bone, and rather lower and more forward than the cardia.

THE INTESTINES.

The intestines form a continued canal from the pylorus, or lower orifice of the stomach, to the anus; and are generally six times the length of the subject to which they belong. They are divided into the large and small intestines—their composition and general structure are similar to that of the stomach. The intestines are furnished with numerous absorbents, called *lacteals.*

THE LIVER.

The liver is the largest viscus of the abdomen. It is situated in the right side—which it occupies entirely—and extends into the left. It is immediately below the diaphragm, and to the right and above the stomach.—The liver is divided into the right and left lobes. The liver is one of the most important glands of the body; and upon its healthy action depends, in a considerable degree, the health of the system. The gall is secreted from the liver, and the gall-bladder is attached to it.

THE PANCREAS.

The pancreas is a glandular body, which has a strong resemblance to the salivary glands. It is situated between the duodenum, or large intestine, and spleen, and is attached to both. It is supposed that the pancreas secretes a fluid similar to the salivary.

THE SPLEEN.

The spleen is a flat body, of an irregular, oblong form. Its common size is four or five inches long, and three or four wide. It is situated in the left hypochondrium, or side, and in contact with the stomach and diaphragm.

THE KIDNEYS.

The kidneys are two glandular bodies which secrete the urine. They are situated in the lumbar region, opposite the last dorsal and first lumbar vertebræ.

THE URETERS.

The ureters are the ducts that convey the urine from

the kidneys to the bladder. They are small, white, elastic tubes, composed of three lamina, or coats.

THE URINARY BLADDER.

The bladder is a large sac, of a muscular and membraneous structure, is situated within the front part of the pelvis, and firmly attached to it.

THE URETHRA

Is the canal, or duct, which conveys the urine off from the bladder.

PART II.

MATERIA MEDICA,

OR

A DESCRIPTION OF MEDICINAL VEGETABLES.

By the term Materia Medica, we understand that part of the medical science, which treats of the nature, composition and relation, of the various substances which are employed in the prevention, cure, and mitigation of diseases; and also the effect of such substances on the human body. It embraces botany, chemistry, and natural history.

Season of collecting Medicinal Vegetables.

Roots should be collected in the spring, before the sap begins to rise, or in the fall, after the top is dead or ripe. Bark may be stripped from the tree or shrub at any time when the sap will prevent it from adhering to the wood. The exterior portion, or ross, should be shaved off, and the bark cut thin for drying.

Medicinal plants should be gathered while in blossom; their virtues, however, are not essentially diminished until they begin to wither.

Seeds should be gathered when fully ripe.

All medicinal vegetables should be dried in the shade. and great care taken that they do not ferment or mould; when thoroughly dried, they should be packed close, and kept from the air, as most vegetables lose a large proportion of their virtues by long exposure to the action of the atmosphere.

Of the proximate principles of Vegetables.

The ultimate analysis of the vegetable substances belonging to the materia medica, is seldom of utility, since we can scarcely ever discover any relation between the composition and medicinal powers of the substance analyzed. The application, therefore, of chemistry to medicinal vegetables, is in a great measure confined to the discrimination of their proximate principles.

These principles are numerous, and of very different kinds, and are not all to be met with in every vegetable, or in every period of vegetation, as some are peculiar to particular plants, or parts of plants, while others are common to almost every plant.

The common proximate principles of vegetables are mostly comprehended under the following heads, viz: *Gum*, *Fecula*, *Gluten*, *Saccharine matter*, *Oil*, *Resin*, *Balsam*, *Tannin*, *Acids*, *Camphor*, *Albumen*, *and Wax*.

Gum is found, more or less pure, in almost all vegetables. It is so abundant in some plants as to be discharged by spontaneous exudation. It is generally impregnated with some other substance. In a pure state, it is inodorous, insipid, glutinous, and soluble in water.

Fecula is a substance approaching in many of its characters to gum. It is soluble in hot water only. It is generally mild and insipid; of a white color.

Starch is the fecula of wheat, corn, and potatoes.

Gluten is usually associated with fecula, and is obtained in the process by which the fecula is separated. It strongly resembles animal gluten—is soluble in alcohol only.

Saccharine matter exists in many vegetable substances, but in combination with mucilage, or extractive matter. It is of a sweet taste—soluble in water and alchohol.

Oil is a common proximate principle of vegetables. It is of two kinds—expressed or fat oil, and distilled volatile or essential oil.

The *expressed*, or *fat oils*, are thick and insipid.—They congeal on exposure to cold—are insoluble in water or alcohol. *Volatile*, or *essential oils*, are obtained by distillation. They are converted into vapor by the heat of boiling water—are so'uble in alcohol only.

Resin.—This principle is in some measure connected with essential oil. The distinguishing properties of a resin, are its existing in a solid state; being insoluble in water, but soluble in alcohol, ether, and oil.

Balsams are resinous juices, with an intermixture generally of essential oil, and containing always a portion of the acid, named benzoic acid.

Tannin.—The important medicinal property of astringency, appears to be dependent, in vegetable substances, on a peculiar principle called tannin. This principle exists in all the vegetable astringents.

Vegetable acids.—The acid formed in the juice and other parts of plants, are not always the same. Not less than seven acids, different from each other, are of vegetable origin, viz: gallic, oxalic, malic, citric, tartaric, benzoic, and acetic.

Camphor is a proximate principle, found in some vegetables, similar in many of its properties to essential oil.

Wax.—Though wax is a substance formed by the bee, yet it is a produce of vegetation.

Albumen.—This principle has been supposed to exist in vegetables, and has been called albumen from its resemblance to the animal principle of that name. It is soluble in cold water, but is coagulated by heat. Like gluten, it is liable to putrefaction.

Extractive matter, is a proximate principle of considerable importance. Its leading character is, that it is soluble equally in pure water and alcohol. This principle is supposed to be the base of what are named *extracts of vegetables.*

A few more component parts might be mentioned, but probably are unnecessary.

Terms of Classification.

Various terms have been introduced into medicine, as indicative both of general and particular kinds of operation, either in health or disease; and those medicines which produce similar operations, have been placed in the same classes or orders. The following are the classes and definitions generally given:—

Narcotics, are substances which diminish the action and powers of the system, without occasioning any sensible evacuation. They have the effects of producing sleep and destroying sensation.

Antispasmodics, are medicines which have the power of allaying irritation and spasms.

Tonics, are those articles which increase the tone of the animal fibre, by which strength is given to the system.

Astringents, are articles which have the power of binding or contracting the fibres of the body.

Emetics, are medicines which excite vomiting, independent of the mere quantity of matter introduced into the stomach.

Cathartics, or *purgatives*, are those medicines which increase the peristaltic motion of the intestines, and thereby produce a preternatural discharge, or operate as physic.

Emmenagogues, are medicines which are capable of promoting the menstrual discharge.

Diuretics, are those medicines which increase the urinary discharge.

Diaphoretics, are those medicines which increase the natural exhalations, or promote moderate perspiration.

Sudorifics, are those medicines which produce copious exhalations, or sweating.

Expectorants, are those medicines which increase the discharge of mucus from the lungs.

Sialagogues, are those medicines which produce a preternatural flow of saliva, from the salivary glands of the mouth and throat.

Epispastics, or *blisters*, are those substances which, when applied to the surface of the body, produce serious or puriform discharges, by exciting a previous state of inflammation.

Rubefacients—substances which, when applied to the skin, stimulate, redden, or inflame it.

Refrigerants—medicines which allay the heat of the body or blood.

Antacids—remedies which obviate acidity (or sourness) of the stomach.

Lithontriptics—medicines which are supposed to possess the power of dissolving urinary concretions in the bladder—as stone, &c.

Escharotics, or caustics, substances which corrode or dissolve the animal solids or flesh.

Anthelmintics—medicines which have the effect of expelling worms from the stomach and bowels.

Demulcents—medicines which obviate and prevent the action of stimulating and acrid substances, by involving them in a mild and viscid substance, which prevents their action on the body.

Diluents—those medicines which increase the fluidity of the blood, or render it lighter and improve the quality.

Emollients—substances which sooth and relax or soften the living fibre.

Alteratives—This term is applied to substances which are found to promote a change in the system favorable to recovery from disease, but not with certainty referable to any other class.

Table of Doses.

As a general rule the following table of doses will be quite sufficient, but much must always be left to the discretion of the prescriber, who alone can judge of the constitution of the patient, and the state of the case.

A person from fourteen to twenty years of age, may take two thirds or three fourths of a dose intended for an adult—from nine to fourteen years, one half—from six to nine, one third—from four to six, one fourth—from two to four, one sixth—from one to two, one tenth—below one year, one twelfth. A woman generally requires a less dose than a man, being generally of weaker constitution.

Apothecaries' Weight.

A pound contains twelve ounces—an ounce eight drachms—a drachm three scruples—a sruple 20 grains.

Measure of Liquids.

A pint contains 16 ounces—an ounce eight drachms. A table-spoonful is about half an ounce—a teaspoonful is one fourth of a table-spoonful. Sixty drops make a teaspoonful.

MEDICINAL VEGETABLES.

In the following description of Medicinal Vegetables, the English name is given first, then the Latin, and lastly the vulgar or common names, which are often numerous. In these descriptions we have endeavored to be brief and comprehensive, as it is always desirable in a work of this kind to keep this object in view. In most instances the class to which the article belongs is given, and the cases in which it is principally employed —but more particular directions for their employment will be found under the head of Pharmacy.

Cayenne Pepper.—*Capsicum annum.*

There are several species of this plant, but their medical properties are nearly the same, except that some are much stronger than others.

This is one of the purest and strongest stimulants with which we are acquainted. It may be used in every form and stage of disease, and acts more powerfully upon the salivary glands than any other substance known. It is carminitive, tonic, diuretic, and emmenagogue. The bright orange colored pepper is best for medical purposes. The dark grey, or brown, is however stronger; this is capsicum nigrum, or African pepper, and is in some cases preferable to the other.

Lobelia Inflata.

This plant is a native of North America, and has a variety of names. It is called lobelia inflata, emetic weed, eye-bright, Indian tobacco, slaber-weed, &c. It is a wild plant, not easily cultivated, and comes up and spreads out like mullen or thistle the first summer; the next season it attains the height of from nine inches to two feet. It branches large, and has numerous capsules about the size of a small bean, with a fringe of fine leaves at the blossom end. The seeds are of a brown color, and very small and numerous; the whole plant is used for medicine. It has, when chewed, rather an insipid taste at first, which soon becomes very acrid and nauseous resembling tobacco. Of the virtues of this plant too much cannot be said. It is a very active emetic, and is perfectly safe in all cases where an emetic is indicated. And from its extensive influence over the animal economy, it is a most effectual remedy in chronic diseases, such as dyspepsia, affections of the liver, diaphragm, spleen, and lungs ; and in all impurities of the blood it may be administered with great advantage. But it should be remembered, that although this plant is very active and stimulating, it is also very volatile, and should be followed by more lasting stimulants.

Bayberry.—*Myrica Cerifera.*

This is a species of myrtle, from which the bayberry tallow, or wax, is obtained. It is a small shrub, growing from two to four feet high, and is most commonly found near the sea shore, and on the banks of lakes and rivers. Its berries grow in bunches close to the body of the shrub, are covered with a white powder, and are about the size of allspice. The leaves which are of a deep green, may be used, but the bark of the root is most important. It is valuable in scrofula, dysentery, jaundice, &c. is astringent and slightly emollient, and for removing canker is excelled by no other article.

Valerian.—*Cyprepedium Pubescens.*

This plant is also called lady's slipper, umbril, nervine, mocasin flower, &c. There are four species of this plant, whose properties are nearly the same, viz.—the yellow, the red, red and white, and white. The yellow grows in swamps where there is not much water, and rises from one to two feet high, with a yellow blossom ; the leaves resemble white hellebore, and the root consists of a thick mat of fine yellow fibres, joined to a main root one fourth of an inch thick. The red grows only on dry land, and has only two leaves that lean over near the ground ; the roots are larger than the yellow. The red, and red and white, resemble each other except in the color of the blossoms, which stand on a single stem rising eight or ten inches.

The root of this plant is sedative, nervine, antispasmodic, and styptic ; it is useful in hysterics, nervous head-aches, epilepsy, tremors, nervous fevers, and in spasmodic affections generally. The dose is a teaspoonful, in warm water or milk.

American Ipecacuanha.—*Apocynum Canabinum.*
Bitter root, Indian hemp, &c.

This root produces a stalk and flowers resembling buckwheat ; the blossom is succeeded by a pod similar to the seed pods of a cabbage, with white down inside ; the stock when broken emits a white substance like milk.

Bitter root is a strong tonic, slightly cathartic and emetic, very useful in cases of indigestion, costiveness and dyspepsia, and is by some used as an errhine in catarrh and colds.

This plant may be found in various parts of the United States, growing in light, sandy soils.

Golden Seal.—*Hydrastis Canadensis.*—Yellow pucoon, Orange root, Yellow root.

This root, which is crooked and wrinkled; is from an eighth to a third of an inch in diameter, with numerous long fibres ; the root is yellow, and the juice pressed out makes a bright yellow stain ; the flowers are flesh, or rose colored, the leaves green, of an oval form, pointed at both ends, and finely indented at the edges ; the stalk rises from eight to twelve inches, and the berry is red and oval. It is a valuable tonic, and at the same time laxative, very useful in dyspepsia and its attendant symptoms, and for correcting the bile, and giving strength and energy to the digestive organs, it is superior to any other article in use.

It is used by some practitioners as a wash for sore and inflamed eyes, sore legs, and as a gargle for sore mouth and throat. Dose, about one third of a teaspoonful.

Bugle.—*Lycopus Virginicus.*
Bugle-wort, Water hoarhound, Archangel.

This is a native of the United States: the seed ripens in September; the leaves are oblong, pointed at the ends and indented at the edges; there is a small burr on each side of the stalk, and close to the leaf, containing two seeds; the blossoms are small and white. It is a good tonic and astringent, and useful in bleeding of the lungs and stomach. It blossoms in July and August. There is another plant resembling this, very bitter, possessing nearly the same qualities; it is also a valuable tonic.

Dose, a teaspoonful; the infusion may also be given.

White Pond Lily.—*Lilium Aquaticum.*

This species of lily is found only in ponds of fresh water. The stem is round and smooth; the leaf is also very smooth, of a bright green, nearly round, and three or four inches in diameter; the flowers are white; the root of a dusky blue on the outside, and covered with a kind of down, which distinguishes it from the yellow lily. It is a powerful astringent, and beneficial in most cases where astringents are indicated. It is particularly useful in removing canker whether external or internal.

Dwarf Elder.—*Sambucus Ebulus.*

This plant bears some resemblance to the sweet elder, particularly the leaves; but the stalk and leaves are smaller, and there are numerous small thorns, like those on gooseberry bushes, near the bottom of the stalk. The flowers are white; the berries are as large as allspice, and are sweet and insipid to the taste, similar to the sweet elder. The whole plant is a mild but very active diuretic, for which it is principally valued. It is useful in dropsy, and diseases of the urinary organs.

Juniper.—*Juniperus.*

This shrub rises from two to four feet high; the leaves slightly resemble the common hemlock, but are sharp and hard. The berries are one fourth of an inch in diameter, of a reddish black color, of aromatic and spicy taste, and chiefly esteemed for medicinal uses. They are a valuable diuretic, a mild stimulant, and useful in colic, and particularly in stranguary and affections of the kidneys.

Boneset.—*Cupatorium Perpoliatum.*

Thorough-wort, Auge weed, Vegetable Antimony.

This is a striking plant, and singular in its appearance. The leaves are long, and sharp pointed ; the stem rises two or three feet high, and is surrounded by the leaf ; the branches rise immediately above the leaves, with a large tuft of white flowers ; the whole plant is covered with a rough down, and is very bitter and nauseous. It is emetic, sudorific, tonic, and cathartic. For an emetic it should be given in a warm infusion ; it is useful in this form to assist other emetics. The leaves may be given with aromatics, in tincture or powder, and are an excellent tonic.

American Saxifrage.—*Saxifragium Communis.*

This plant grows on light soils, near rivers, and rises from twelve to eighteen inches high ; the leaves are of a beautiful deep green, resembling those of the sweet elder, with fine indentations at the edges ; the stalk rises above the leaves, and branches like caraway, with a tuft of small yellow blossoms ; the seed are small and of a dark brown ; the roots are from one to three inches long, brown on the outside, of a light yellow within, and from one fourth to one eighth of an inch thick. This plant is a powerful sudorific, or sweating medicine. It is also diuretic and sialagogue.

White Snake Root.—*Actea Racemosa.*

This plant rises from two to four feet high, with a smooth square stalk ; the leaves are oval at the stem, and pointed at the end, with large indentations at the edges, and of a dark green color ; The flowers are white, and stand in a regular tuft on the top of the stem ; the roots are very numerous, and very small fibres are attached to a small hard root, of a dark brown color ; it has a warm aromatic taste. The remedial properties of the roots of this plant are sudorific and diuretic. It is useful in fevers generally, in infusion or powder.

Poplar.—*Liriodendron Tulipifera.*

There are several species of the poplar, but the black is best for medicine. The bark towards the root is black and rough ; there are tags which hang on until the leaves put out ; the leaves are always in motion when there is any wind, which gives it the name of quaking asp.

The bark is a valuable tonic, perhaps equal to any which this country affords, for dyspepsia, and all complaints of the stomach and bowels ; it is also a good alterative. It may be administered in powder, infusion, or extract, alone, or combined with other articles. It is highly recommended in affections of the liver.

Fir Balsam.—*Pinus Balsamea.*

This balsam is obtained from the fir tree. It is a valuable medicine, applied externally or internally ; for internal soreness occasioned by strains or debility it is a superior remedy ; it is a valuable ingredient in salves, and also a mild emmenagogue.

Vervine.—*Verbena hastata.*
Life of man, Fever root.

There are two kinds of vervine, blue and white ; it grows by the side of brooks and roads, and rises three or four feet high, with long branches ; the flowers and seed lie close to the stalk ; the top resembles the seed stalk of the common plantain ; the leaves are large, of a deep green, and largely indented at the edges ; the roots are of fine fibres and long. This plant is a good expectorant and sudorific ; the root is tonic, alterative, and emmenagogue, and is much used by some practitioners in pulmonary consumption.

Skullcap.—*Scutellaria Lateriflora.*

Mad weed. Hood-wort, Blue Pimpernell.

This herb rises with a square hollow stem, from one to three feet high—one eighth or fourth of an inch in diameter. The leaves are an inch long, oval at the stem, and pointed at the other end. The blossoms small, single, and blue. The seed-bowls are of a singular shape, opening like a clam shell. The upper part has a sharp ridge running across it. The seeds are small, white, and hard. The medical properties of this plant are—tonic, nervine, and antispasmodic. It is used in the St. Vitus' dance, tetanus, tremors, convulsions, and hydrophobia; in which disease it is recommended by some practitioners as a sovreign remedy. This is the medicine so extensively used by the Vanderesveers in the cure of hydrophobia in men and beasts. The dose of the powder is a large teaspoonfull. It may be given freely in the infusion.

Hoarhound.—*Marrubium vulgare.*

Hoarhound is a stimulant, pectoral tonic, emmenagogue, and antispasmodic—valuable in colds, coughs, and pulmonary diseases generally.

Skunk Cabbage.—*Ictodes fœtida.*

The appearance of this plant is noble; the leaves are large, resembling cabbage, but of a light green; the seed are contained in a rough, spongy bulb, which stands on a very short stem in the centre of the plant, and are brown when ripe—one third of an inch thick, irregularly round. The whole plant possesses a very fetid smell, resembling that of assafœtida, or the odor thrown off by the skunk. The root of this plant is a very strong antispasmodic, expoctorant, and nervine. It is used with great success in asthma, croup, and hysterics, in which last disease it is particularly useful; and also in tusis senales, or that kind of cough which frequently attends old persons without much expectoration.

Slippery Elm.—*Elmus fulva.*

The inside bark of this tree is an article of extraordinary value. Its medical properties are those of a demulcent, diuretic, expectorant, emolient, and refrigerent—useful in urinary and bowel complaints, stranguary, sore throat, catarrh, pleurisy, inflammation of the stomach, bowels, and lungs; scurvy, herpes, inveterate eruptions of the skin; for an external application in the form of a poultice, it is not surpassed by any known production of the world; also for ulcers, burns, tumors, scabs, thrush, and particularly for gun-shot wounds. It is easily distinguished from the other kinds of elm, by the mucilaginous substance contained in the bark.

Black Alder.—*Prinos verticillatus.*

Tag alder, Swamp alder.

This species of alder grows in wet land near streams of water; rises ten or fifteen feet high, in clusters; the boughs are covered with smooth tags in the spring. Alder is useful in all impurities of the blood, particularly in scrofulous and herpetic affections.

Dandelion.—*Leontodon taraxacum.*

The dandelion is a popular remedy for diseases of the liver and spleen, and is highly beneficial in jaundice and hypochondria. It is diuretic, deabstruant, and tonic.

Prickly Ash.—*Zanthoxylum fraxineum.*

This is a beautiful tree, rising fifteen or twenty feet high; the limbs are furnished with numerous prickles resembling those of the large black-berry brier; the bark is thin and externally yellowish; white internally; taste warm and aromatic, exciting a copious discharge of saliva, or spittle; the berries grow in clusters on the top of the branches; are small, black, or deep blue, enclosed in a grey shell. The bark is an energetic stimulant, and diaphoretic; useful in chronic rheumatism; the berries are a good tonic, and aperient; are used in dyspepsia.

Blood root.—*Sanguinaria Canadensis.*

The leaves of this plant are of a light green, irregularly round; the root is about one third of an inch thick, several roots connecting together; when broken, a reddish, orange-colored juice is discharged abundantly.—Blood root is emetic, cathartic, emmenagogue, sialagogue, and lithontriptic; also strongly diuretic, caustic, and an excellent errhine; it is particularly useful in form of snuff for catarrh, &c.

Comfrey.—*Symphitum.*

Comfrey is a domestic plant; the leaves resemble the mullen, but are of a darker green; the blossoms are small and white; the root is black outside, and white within; of an insipid mucilaginous taste; it is demulcent and astringent; used in dyssentery, pulmonary irritation, and consumption.

Tanzy.—*Tanacetum.*

Tanzy is a stimulating emmenagogue, and tonic; useful in hysterics and dropsy; also in diseases of the urinary organs, it is used with success.

Plantain.—*Plantago.*

The plantain is found in wood-yards and gardens, and by the sides of roads; the leaves are four or five inches long, and ribbed on the under side; the seed-stalks rise from six to eighteen inches; the seeds lie close to the stalk, and nearly cover it for one quarter of the length at the top. It is undoubtedly a great counter poison, and of extraordinary value for curing the bite of spiders and venomous serpents, for which purpose it may be combined with hoarhound and given in such quantities as the stomach can bear, and applied to the wound.

Witch Hazel.—*Hamamelis Virginica.*

This shrub rises from ten to fifteen feet high, in irregular clusters, like alder. The blossoms remain during the winter; they are irregular yellow tags, closely attached to the limbs. The decoction of the leaves, or bark, is valuable for removing canker, and an excellent application for the piles, prolapsus of the bowels, &c.

Butternut.—*Juglans cincrea.*

The extract of the bark acts as a cathartic, without occasioning any heat or irritation; taken in large doses, it will operate as an emetic; it is a good tonic in very small doses.

Bitter-Sweet.—*Solanum Dulcamara.*

Bitter-Sweet is a woody vine, resembling the grape, but smooth and gray; the berries are light red; the root is reddish yellow. The bark of the root is discutient, from which an ointment may be made for herpetic diseases, and removing corns and callouses.

Ox Balm.—*Piunkum.*

Hard Root, Toad Root.

The stalk of the ox balm is square and smooth; rises three feet high; the leaves are from four to six inches long, and from three to four wide; the flowers are small and single; stand along near the top of the stalk and branches; of a strong, aromatic smell; the whole plant is pale green. The root is an irregular oval, with knots of various shapes and sizes; the whole root is half as large as a man's fist; brown externally, and hard; the root of this plant is a powerful lithontriptic, discutient, and deobstruent; very valuable for removing gravel and other substances from the bladder and kidneys, and for almost all diseases to which the urianry organs are subject; also for removing glandular and other swellings, but should not be applied where there is a tendency to suppuration; it is of great utility in night sweats.

Gentian.—*Gentiana lutea.*

Gentian, Gensing, &c.

Gentian is generally found on dry, ledgy land, where the soil is light and rich; the stalk rises three feet high; is round and rather rough; the leaves are from five to seven inches long, and from three to five inches wide. The fruit resembles that of the red thorn; are a pale orange color; the seed are covered with sharp, white hairs, and are hard, like the thorn seed. The roots are from one third to half an inch thick; they are one or two feet long; the bark of the root is very thick and tender; the inner part hard and tough. Gentian is an invaluable medicine in diseases of every species, but particularly in coughs and consumption; it is also a good stomachic and tonic.

Red Raspberry.—*Rubus strigusosus.*

The leaves of this plant are astringent, and useful in dysentery; in removing canker from any part of the system; and in healing relaxations of any of the internal organs.

Queen of the Meadow.—*Spiræa ulmaria.*

Queen of the Meadow flourishes best on rich bottom land, near streams of water; the stalks are hollow and round, rising from four to six feet high; crowned with a tuft of red blossoms, of an inferior appearance. The leaves are six or eight inches long, and two wide; rather rough. The root is composed of numerous brown fibres, an eighth of an inch thick; there are numerous short, red stripes on the stalk. The root of this plant is an excellent diuretic; used with great success in suppression of urine, inflammation of the kidneys, and indiscriminately where diuretics are indicated.

Common Hemlock.—*Pinus Canadensus.*

The inner bark of the hemlock is an excellent astringent; good to remove canker, and in relaxations of the bowels, &c. The distilled oil is a valuable application for quinzy and swelled throat; the gum forms an excellent plaster for lumbago and rheumatism; the leaves are a good sudorific.

Mandrake.—*Podophyllum peltatum.*

The medical properties of this plant are purgative, deobstruent, antibillious, anthelmintic, hydrogogue, and antidyspeptic. A popular writer, speaking of this root, says there is no article which answers better the purposes of jalap, aloes, and rhubarb, than the mandrake, or is more mild in its operation. Combined with lobelia, it is an excellent cathartic in most cases where a cathartic is indicated, and particularly for removing worms.

Common Sumach.—*Rhus tiphinum.*

Sumach bark, of the root, is used in decoction for falling of the bowels; and mixed with elm or Indian meal, forms a valuable poultice. The infusion of the berries makes an excellent gargle for sore throat and mouth.

Balmony.

This herb grows on wet land, near streams of water; it is about the size of peppermint; has a square stalk, and a white blossom, resembling a snake's head with the mouth open. It is tonic and antibilious, and calculated to restore the appetite and digestive powers.

English Saxifrage.—*Pimpinelli Saxifragium.*

This plant is a native of Europe, but easily cultivated in our gardens. It rises from two to three feet high; the leaves are a deep bright green, sharply indented at the edges; the stalk is from a third to half an inch in diameter, and rises above the leaves, with a bunch of white blossoms, resembling caraway, but larger. The root slightly resembles the parsnip near the top, and branches out toward the bottom. The tincture of the root of this plant, in gin, is one of the most powerful diuretics that is to be found in the whole materia medica; it is of great value in dropsy of the chest and abdomen, and in incontinence of urine.

Blue Scabish.

Frost-weed, Squaw-weed, Cocash.

This plant grows on wet, boggy land; the stalks are round, and three feet in height; the leaves four to six inches long, and one to two wide; the blossoms are blue, and continue until killed by the frost; the roots are small, brown, and of a warm aromatic taste. Scabish is useful in removing canker; the infusion makes a good wash for sore mouth and throat, and the strong decoction may be taken with advantage in rheumatism.

Peach Tree.

The bark and leaves of the peach tree are a good tonic, but the kernel or meat of the stone is a superior article; highly beneficial in dyspepsia, or weakness of the stomach. The wild black cherry stones, and bitter almonds, possess nearly the same qualities.

Dragon Turnip.—*Arum Triphillum.*

Wild Turnip, Pepper Turnip, Wake-Robin, March Turnip.

This plant grows from one to two feet high. It has three leaves at the end of a stem; the seed stock is enclosed in a sheath, which when open resembles a flower; the berries form a compact bunch, of a bright red; the root is round and flattened, of an acrid, pungent, and caustic taste, an expectorant, and a powerful discutient. A poultice of the green plant, with elm or meal, is a good application for scrofulous and other swellings; an ointment of the root, with lard, is a good application in tinca capitis, or scalded head; it may be used with advantage in coughs and colics, in doses of a teaspoonful or less. In autumn there may be found small sets, or turnips, under the old one, which, when pulverized, form a mild and valuable caustic.

Spikenard.—*Aralia Racemosa.*

Spikenard rises three feet high, with large branches, and large clusters of black berries; the roots are of the size of a man's finger, long and brown, of a warm, balsamic, sweetish taste, and valuable in decoction for coughs and colds; it is also a good tonic and restorative; the tincture of the berries is used for rheumatism.

Rose Willow.—*Cornus Sericea.*

Red Rod, Red Willow.

This shrub grows near streams of water; the young branches are very smooth, and of a beautiful red; the infusion forms an excellent eye-water.

Solomon Seal.—*Convallaria Multiflora.*

This plant rises from six inches to three feet, according to the soil on which it grows; the stalk is smooth, and the leaves oval, thin, and ribbed; the flowers are white; berries black, round and single, hanging by a single stem on each side the stalk; the root is white and tender; it is astringent, demulcent and restorative, and is used in decoction or syrup, for fluor albus immoderate flow of the menses, &c.

Cranebill..—*Geranium Maculatum.*

This plant rises one or two feet high; the leaves are irregular, with several joints; flowers of a lilac or rose color; root rough, and dark brown; the root, when boiled in milk, proves efficacious in cholera infantum, that kind of diarrhœa to which young children are subject; also in sore throat and mouth, and bleeding at the stomach and lungs.

Sassafras.—*Laurus Sassafras.*

The bark is stimulating and attenuating; good in rheumatism and dysentery; the pith of the young branches infused in cold water is used in inflammation of the eyes, and dysentery, and if drank for some time, is a sovereign remedy for the piles.

Spear-mint.—*Mentha Viridis.*

Spear-mint is diuretic, sudorific, and anti-emetic; the infusion drank allays the irritability of the stomach, and stops vomiting.

Dragon's Claw.—*Pterisfora Andromada.*

Fever Root.

This plant rises from six to ten inches; the blossoms are small and yellow; the seed bowls hang over by a single stem; the stalk has a kind of husk; the roots form a compact cluster, or bunch; they are abont as large as cloves, and are very tender; slightly attached to the stalk; the root is diaphoretic and sudorific.

Yellow Dock.—*Rumex Crispus.*

This species of dock grows plenty in this country; the stalk rises two feet; the upper part is covered with seed in autumn; the leaves are from four to ten inches long, and two wide. The root is yellow and branching.—There is another species of dock that resembles this, but the leaves are wider and streaked with red. The yellow dock is useful in removing cancerous, scrofulous, and other taints from the system; it is an alterative of great value.

Whipsiwog.—*Fox tail, Horse tail, Fire weed.*

This plant grows abundantly on land that has been ploughed or cleared but one or two years. It rises from two to six feet high, with a branching, bushy top. The blossoms are succeeded by a kind of chaff, or down; the leaves are long and narrow; the whole plant is rough. This is one of the most powerful and yet mild styptics which the earth affords. It may be used in infusion or decoction. The expressed juice, or distilled oil, (which it affords abundantly by distillation,) in all effusions of blood from wounds or other causes, whether external or internal, is the most powerful, and should be combined with alcohol to form an essence for internal use. It is also antidysenteric, and used with advantage in diarrhœa and relaxation of the bowels.

Red Mulberry.—*Morus Rubra, Scotch Cap.*

This species of mulberry resembles the raspberry in the fruit and bush, but is larger and more woody. The leaves are nearly as large as a man's hand, with three long points. The root is half an inch thick, or less; long and hard, with numerous branches. The root is used with considerable success in diabetes, prolapsus of the bladder, urethra, and relaxations of the urinary organs generally.

Cleavers.—*Garlium Aparvine.*

This is a kind of joint-grass. The stalk is square; the corners are rough, like a sickle; there are small leaves that put out at every joint, half an inch long, and very narrow. The blossoms are small, white, and very numerous. It is a valuable diuretic and emmenagogue; very usseful in some cases of female debility. The infusion should be used nearly cold, as boiling injures its medicinal properties.

Ginger.—*Amomum Zingiber.*

Ginger is a warm, aromatic stimulant, and sudorific; very useful in colds, flatulent colics, laxity and debility of the intestines. It promotes circulation, and relieves pain.

Myrrh.—*Amyris Katap.*

Myrrh is a gummy, resinous, concrete substance, obtained from a tree which grows in Arabia Felix, and

Abyssinia, near the Red Sea. The best myrrh is somewhat transparent, brown, or reddish yellow, and of a pungent, bitter taste. It is used internally as a stimulant, antiseptic, and emmenagogue; externally, as a detergent wash in foul ulcers. It powerfully resists putrefaction and gangrene.

Aloes.—*Aloe Spricata.*

There are several species of aloes, but the socotorine is the best. It is a warm, stimulating purgative, and emmenagogue. If given in large doses, it excites irritation of the intestines, producing piles and other unpleasant symptoms; given in small doses, it is a good tonic, and assists digestion.

Dog Mackymoose.—*Indian tobacco tree.*

This shrub, or tree, rises from eight to twelve feet, with a branching top. The bark is dark brown, and nearly smooth. The leaves are oval at the stem, and pointed at the other end; two inches long, and ribbed on the under side. The flowers are white, and the berries very numerous. They are green, then red; and when ripe, a dark blue; the size of small peas. The bark of this tree is a good alterative, useful in scrofulous, herpetic, and all impurities of the blood.

Spotted Maple.—*Cancer Maple.*

This tree rises ten or fifteen feet. The bark is spotted, or greyish green and white. The leaves resemble the large soft maple, as does also the seed, which it produces abundantly. The medical properties are much the same as the mackymoose; used for cancers.

Wild Lettuce.

This is a small plant. The leaves are as large as a cent; of a light green. They grow on a stem, like the winter-green. The seed-stalk rises from three to six inches; the blossoms are small and white. The lettuce is used for sore mouth. The extract, with other articles, form an excellent salve.

Wood Sorrel, Sheep Sorrel, &c.

This plant grows from three to six inches high. The leaves are small and round, the blossoms yellow, and rather a pale green. From this species of sorrel, a valuable plaster is made for the cure of cancers.

Poke, Scoke, Pigeon Berry, Garget Root.

Poke is very common in the United States on new land, by road sides, and by the side of old logs. It rises from three to six feet high. The stalks are of a reddish color, with large branches. The leaves are large. The berries grow in large clusters, of a reddish blue or black. When ripe, they are used in gin for the dysentery, and enter into ointments. The root, roasted in embers, forms a powerful poultice.

White Hellebore.—*Helleborus*

Bear Weed, Itch Weed.

This plant is found in moist land, near streams of water. It is the first plant that comes up in the spring, and grows two feet high with a round stalk. The leaves are from six to ten inches long, and three or four wide. The roots are numerous, white, and long, resembling the skunk cabbage, but smaller. The decoction of the root is used for poultices, and the powder in snuff.

Fennel.—*Anethum Fœniculum.*

Fennel is a garden plant, used in flatulence, indigestion, weakness, pain in the breast, and cholic—for children.

Virginia Snake Root.—*Aristolochia serpentaria.*

The root is knotty, with long, small fibres, which are yellow when fresh, and brown when dry. The stalks are small and slender, bearing from three to seven leaves, and from one to three flowers. The leaves are heart-shaped at the stem, and pointed at the other end; smooth, and of a pale green; it is found at the shops, the whole plant dried. It grows in shady woods, from Massachusetts to Florida, but most abundant in the Cumberland and Alleghany Mountains. It is diaphoretic, tonic, anodyne, cordial, antispasmodic, a powerful stimulant, and counter-poison.

Jalap.—*Convolvulus Jalappa.*

This plant is a native of Mexico and Vera Cruz. It is an active cathartic, and produces very little griping or irritation of the stomach or bowels.

Alexandria Senna.—*Cassia Senna.*

Senna is a very useful cathartic and anthelmintic. and combined with other articles, is an excellent remedy for worms.

Gamboge.—*Garcinia Gambogia.*

The tree that furnishes the gamboge is of middle size, and grows wild in the kingdoms of Siam and Ceylon. The gum is obtained by incision, from which the juice exudes. It is a powerful emetic and cathartic, if given in large doses; in small doses, it acts as a mild laxative. Gamboge is found, in commerce, in rolls of various sizes, of a yellow color.

Garden Anise-seed.—*Pimpinella Anisum.*

The properties of anise, are similar to those of fennel. The seed is carminative and pectoral; it is useful in dyspepsia, and flatulent affections incident to children.

Seneca Snake root.—*Polygala Senega.*

This plant is found in Pennsylvania and Virginia.—The stem grows from six to ten inches high. The leaves are long and sharp pointed. The root is from the size of a quill to that of the finger; its odor is weak and nauseous. The bark is gray; the taste is sweet, then acrid and bitter.

Rhubarb.—*Rheum Palmatum.*

Rhubarb is a native of China and Tartary, but is cultivated in Europe and America. The stalk rises from two to four feet high. The leaves are very large and irregular; the root is of various forms. It is a valuable and singular cathartic, differing from all others. It first operates by evacuating the intestinal canal, and then gently astringing or restoring the tone of it. Upon this singular combination of properties, (purgative and astringent,) depends its utility in dysenteries and diarrhœa. In cholera, its medicinal properties are heightened. It is also very valuable combined with soda, in neutralizing the acidity of the stomach.

Carolina Pink.—*Spigelia Marilandica.*

The stems are numerous; from one to two feet high; square, and of a purplish color; leaves few opposite on the stalk. The flowers are of a beautiful carmine color. The root consists of a number of fine, black fibres, forming together a large bunch. This article possesses surprising anthelmintic, or vermifuge properties, and is a very popular remedy for worms. It should be combined with, or followed by, some cathartic, as senna or mandrake. Given in large doses, it has the effect of narcotics, producing drowsiness, acceleration of the pulse, mental derangement, &c.

Celedine—(*Chelidonium.*)

This is a garden plant. It is luxuriant with irregular leaves; small, yellow blossoms. When the stalk is broken, it emits a reddish or yellowish fluid. The leaves simmered in butter, form a valuable salve.

PART III.

ON PHARMACY,

OR THE PREPARATION OF MEDICINES.

Pharmacy is that branch of the medical science, which teaches the art of preparing and combining remedies for the treatment of diseases.

POWDERS.

Powders are the most natural and simple form in which medicines can be administered, as their virtues are not impaired by passing through the process of pulverization. All powders should be kept in glass or stone vessels, closely stopped, and excluded from the light, otherwise their virtues may be impaired.

1. *Alterative Powders.*

Take bayberry bark one pound, hemlock bark eight ounces, cayenne pepper two ounces, ginger eight ounces, white pond lily four ounces, and cloves two ounces; mix them well together and they are fit for use.

Dose—a teasppoonful is a medium dose.

Use—These powders may be given in all cases and stages of diseases to which men, women and children are subject. They answer the general purposes of an alterative to establish perspiration, equalize circulation, and remove obstructions, from cold or other causes.

Poplar bark is a useful ingredient in the above, where a tonic is required.

2. *Cough Powder.*

Take of hoarhound two ounces, skunk cabbage four ounces, wild turnip one ounce, boneset one ounce, lobelia leaves one ounce, gentian one ounce, valerian one ounce, and cayenne pepper one ounce, thoroughly mixed.

Dose—one teaspoonful for an adult, or half a teaspoonful or less for a child of two years.

Use—for cough occasioned by cold, hooping-cough, inflammation of the lungs, &c.

3. *Emetic Powder.*

Take of lobelia two ounces, valerian one ounce; pulverize and mix.

Dose—from one to two teaspoonfuls.

Use—This emetic may be given in most cases where an emetic is proper; it should be given in half a teacupful of warm water, with two teaspoonfuls of vegetable elixir; this quantity should be given once in thirty or forty minutes, until it operates. If it should occasion pain in the stomach, give the vegetable elixir to warm the stomach, and a solution of soda, sal eratus, or pearlash, to neutralize the acid, or sourness. This emetic should generally be accompanied with an injection to remove canker from the bowels, and the steam bath, to raise a perspiration.

4. *Cephalic Snuff.*

Take of bayberry bark one ounce, blood root one ounce; mix. Used for catarrh, head-ache and polypus.

5. *Compound Powder of Mandrake.*

Take of mandrake one ounce, spear-mint one ounce, soda half an ounce.

Use—for diseases of the liver, dyspepsia, &c.

SYRUPS.

Syrups are liquids, containing the properties of certain vegetables in a very concentrated state. They are prepared by boiling the ingredients until their strength is extracted, and much of the watery portion evaporated; then adding a sufficient quantity of clarified sugar to prevent fermentation.

In consequence of the oléaginous and other peculiar

properties contained in most vegetables, water is not sufficient to extract their virtues, and it is necessary to use spirits. The two menstruums combined answer the purpose admirably; after the alcohol has extracted the component parts of the vegetables, it is evaporated by boiling, when no danger need be apprehended from its stimulating effects.

6. *Alterative Syrup.*

Take of dandelion root one pound, gentian one pound, spotted maple bark one pound, dog mackamoose bark one pound, burdock root one pound, yellow dock root one pound, white ash bark one pound, bitter root one fourth of a pound, mandrake root one fourth of a pound, white snake root one pound; add one gallon spirits and one gallon water; boil half an hour; pour off, add water, and boil until the strength of the ingredients are obtained; then boil the whole to three gallons; then strain it, and add six pounds sugar; boil and skim it; let it settle, and bottle for use.

Dose.—A wine glass full three times a day, before eating.

Use.—This syrup possesses extraordinary virtues, and is used with remarkable success in a great variety of diseases. In syphilis, or venereal; chronic inflammation of the liver; scrofula, in all its various forms; white swellings; rickets; salt rheum, or herpes; and in almost every taint of the system, it acts powerfully upon the secretions and excretions, and is undoubtedly superior to Swaim's celebrated Panacea.

7. *Diuretic Syrup.*

Take of dwarf elder one pound, anise-seed half a pound, senna half a pound, English saxifrage two ounces, ox balm one pound, juniper eight ounces, mandrake root four ounces, queen of the meadow roots two pounds, sassafras bark of the root one pound, gentian eight ounces, valerian eight ounces, lobelia one ounce; obtain the strength as above; boil to one gallon; add two pounds sugar; strain, settle, and bottle for use.

Dose.—A wine glass full three or four times a day.

Use.—This syrup is useful in all cases of dropsy, chronic inflammation of the kidneys, &c.

8. *Antispasmodic Syrup.*

Take of skunk cabbage seed four ounces, burdock seed four ounces, valerian four ounces, bayberry bark four ounces, skull-cap four ounces, cayenne pepper one ounce; add one gallon water; boil to one quart; strain it, and add one pound loaf sugar.

Dose.—For an adult, a tablespoonful; for a child one year old, a teaspoonful.

Use.—This syrup is a valuable antispasmodic, and may be administered in hysterics, convulsions, and spasmodic affections generally—both as a remedy and preventative in irritable and nervous habits.

9. *Tonic Syrup.*

Take of garden piony root one pound, Peruvian bark four ounces, bayberry bark eight ounces, Virginia snake root four ounces; extract the strength; boil to two quarts; add four pounds loaf sugar.

Dose.—From one to three tablespoonfuls.

Use.—To be given as a tonic when a patient is recovering from fever, &c.

10. *Scrofulous Syrup*

Take of bayberry bark one pound, sarsaparilla six pounds, sweet elder flowers two pounds, guaiacum shavings three pounds, sassafras root two pounds; add spirits and water, and boil repeatedly until the strength is obtained; boil to two gallons; strain it, and add ten pounds sugar; boil and settle, and it is fit for use.

Dose.—A wine glass full three times a day.

Use.—This is a very good alterative, given in scrofula and impurities of the blood generally, and is by some practitioners considered preferable to all others of this class.

11. *Pulmonary Syrup*

Take of liverwort eight ounces, Solomon seal one pound, skunk cabbage one pound, blood root four ounces, water hoarhound one pound; boil until the strength is obtained; strain and boil to two gallons; add ten lbs. honey; settle and bottle for use.

Dose.—From half to a wine glass full.

Use.—This syrup is used in every variety of pulmonary diseases, particularly in bleeding of the lungs, and asthmatic affections.

12. *White Poppy Syrup.*

Take of the capsules, or pods of white poppies, eight ounces, water one pint; infuse them twelve hours; then boil fifteen minutes; then strain, and add sufficient sugar to preserve it.

Dose.—From ten to fifteen drops.

Use.—This syrup forms a good anodyne for infants, as it contains less of the narcotic properties of the poppy than when prepared in spirits. It relieves pain, and causes sleep, similar in its effects to paregoric.

CORDIALS.

By this class of medicines, we understand those preparations containing the virtues of various vegetables, prepared similar to common cordials. After the decoction of the articles which compose the cordial are sufficiently concentrated, sugar, mucilage, spirits, honey, &c. are added to make them more agreeable to the taste, and mild in their operation.

13. *Pulmonary Cordial.*

Take of gentian root two ounces, elecampane two ounces, dandelion flowers one ounce, lobelia herb one ounce, hoarhound two ounces, valerian one ounce, skunk cabbage two ounces, sweet wine two quarts, honey two pounds, loaf sugar two pounds, and one calf's pluck cut fine. Put these articles into a stone jar; cover it with a dough crust an inch thick; secure the crust in such a manner that no steam can escape; then bake it for two hours in an oven of higher temperature than is necessary to bake bread; then strain it, pressing out all the juice that can be obtained, and bottle it for use. The whole pluck should be used, the fatty substance excepted.

Dose.—From a teaspoonful to a tablespoonful.

Use.—This cordial is highly useful in the treatment of pulmonary diseases generally, and particularly in phthisis pulmonalis, or consumption; and for all diseases of the lungs not attended with acute inflammation. The liver, lights, heart, and gall should be used.

14. *Restorative Cordial.*

Take of comfrey root one pound, Solomon seal one pound, spikenard one pound, colombo root eight ounces, gentian eight ounces, camomile flowers four ounces, water two gallons; infuse for twelve hours at blood heat; then strain, and add two qts. of wine or matheglin.

Dose.—A wine-glass full, or less, two or three times a day.

Use.—This is a very useful tonic in all cases of debility or weakness, when the system is in a situation to bear strengthening; in incipient consumption, fluor albus, &c.

15. *Expectorant Cordial.*

Take of comfrey one pound, elecampane one pound, hoarhound one pound, skunk cabbage eight ounces, spikenard one pound, lobelia one ounce; boil the whole repeatedly until the strength is obtained; then strain it; boil to two gallons; then add eight pounds loaf sugar, four pounds honey, and four eggs; boil and skim it, and bottle for use.

Dose.—From half to a wine-glass full, three or four times a day.

Use.—This cordial is useful in chronic inflammation of the lungs, coughs of long standing, and consumption, and assists breathing and expectoration. It does not increase the circulation, and may therefore be used with perfect safety.

16. *Antidysenteric Cordial.*

Take of black birch bark one pound, bayberry bark one pound, poplar bark one pound, bitter almonds one pound, water two gallons ; boil to one gallon and a half; then add half a gallon cogniac brandy, and four pounds loaf sugar.

Dose.—A wine-glass full three times a day, for an adult.

Use.—This is an excellent tonic and astringent, for dysentery and diarrhœa of long standing.

Drops.

Drops include those remedies, which, from their strength or active properties, require to be given in very minute doses ; the dose being usually graduated by the number to be administered. Great care or caution is necessary in giving this class of medicines, as mistakes are more liable to be made than in some other forms.—Phials, containing drops, should always be kept corked, that their strength may not be increased by evaporation, or their virtue lost.

17. *Bateman's Drops.*

Take of fennel seed four ounces, anise seed two ounces, Virginia snake root two ounces, red sanders one ounce, opium one fourth ounce, rum one gallon ; put the whole into a stone jug after pulverizing ; shake it once a day for a week ; it is then fit for use.

Dose.—From ten drops to a teaspoonful.

Use.—These drops are anodyne and carminative ; they ease pain, produce sleep, and are useful with the vegetable elixir in cholera morbus, diarrhœa, &c.

18. *Diuretic Drops.*

Take of sweet spirits of nitre two ounces, oil of

almonds two ounces, balsam copaiba one ounce, spirits of turpentine half an ounce, camphor one eighth ounce.

Dose.—From ten to twenty drops three times a day, in mucilage of gum Arabia or slippery elm.

19. *Hydragogue Drops.*

Take of dwarf elder berries one gill, Holland gin one pint; let it stand, and shake it once a day until the berries are dissolved; then strain and keep it corked.

Dose.—From half a teaspoonful to two spoonfulls.

Use.—These drops possess very active properties, and are used with extraordinary success in dropsy of the thorax and abdomen; they are an excellent diuretic, and may be given in inflammation of the kidneys and stranguary, and in all cases where a diuretic is required.

20. *Cough Drops.*

Take oil of anise one ounce, oil of almonds one ounce, balsam fir one ounce, tincture of balsam tolu one ounce, wine one ounce; shake the whole together until thoroughly incorporated.

Dose.—Fifteen to twenty drops in mucilage, or tea.

Use.—These drops may be given in most cases of cough; they assist breathing and expectoration.

21. *Carminative Drops*

Take of angelica four ounces, valerian two ounces, calamus half an ounce, anise seed one ounce, fennel seed one ounce, dill seed one ounce, catnip leaves or blossoms one ounce, motherwort one ounce; infuse the whole in two quarts of brandy for twelve hours, in moderate heat; then strain it and add one pound loaf sugar.

Dose.—For a child, from ten to forty drops; for an adult, a teaspoonful.

Use.—It eases pain, causes perspiration, sleep, &c. good for restless children, and in hysterics and nervous affections.

22. *Whitwith's Drops.*

Take of camphor one ounce, oil origanum six ounces, spirits of turpentine half an ounce, alcohol one quart; mix and shake daily for one week.

Dose.—Twenty-five drops in wine or sweetened water.

Use.—This preparation is useful as a stimulant, and may be applied externally in rheumatism and other painful affections.

23. *Balsam of Honey.*

Take of balsam tolu two ounces, balsam fir two ounces, opium one ounce; dissolve them in one quart alcohol.

Dose.—From half to a teaspoonful two or three times a day.

Use.—This preparation is useful in pulmonary diseases generally; it allays irritation and inflammation. This is the celebrated balsam of honey which is sold at the shops.

24. *Tooth-ache Drops.*

Take of the oil of sassafras one ounce, oil of cloves one ounce, oil of summer-savory one ounce, oil of cedar one ounce; mix; dip a piece of lint in the drops, and put it in the tooth; either of the above ingredients may be used alone.

DECOCTIONS.

Decoctions are certain preparations of medicines, made by boiling substances in water, for a considerable time. Where we wish to administer the active properties of any plant in small volume in the form of drinks, decoctions are very useful; some vegetables, however, lose their efficacy by long boiling, and are given best in some other form.

25. *Diurctic Decoctions.*

Take of the queen of the meadow two ounces, milkweed two ounces, juniper berries two ounces, dwarf elder root two ounces, ox balm four ounces, spikenard two ounces; boil; make a strong decoction.

Dose, from a gill to half a pint.

Useful in dropsies, stranguary, affections of the kidneys, gravel, &c. It is strongly diuretic.

FOMENTATIONS.

Fomentations are usually composed of several bitter herbs, and are useful in removing pain and inflammation, by taking off tension and spasm, or to brace and restore the tone and vigor of those parts to which they are applied.

The first of these intentions may generally be answered by warm fomentations, and the second by those that are cold. This class of medicines are valuable in a great variety of diseases.

26. *Lobelia Fomentations.*

Take of lobelia seed, pulverized, one ounce, vinegar one pint; mix.

Use.—This fomentation is of great value in external inflammation, particularly in inflammation of the head or brain; in which disease it exceeds all others. It should be applied cold.

27. *Bitter Fomentation.*

Take of hops one ounce, tanzy one ounce, wormwood one ounce, hoarhound one ounce, catnip one ounce; make a strong decoction by boiling in equal parts of vinegar and water. This fomentation will be found very efficacious in removing pain and inflammation caused by sprains, dislocation, and contusions.

28. *Stimulating Fomentation.*

Take of lobelia one ounce, cayenne pepper two ounces, mustard seed two ounces, spirits two quarts. This is an excellent application in paralytic affections, cold and numbness of the limbs, and other parts.

29. *Mint Fomentation.*

Take of fresh spear-mint three ounces, spirits half a pint; simmer ten minutes.

Use.—This fomentation, applied to the stomach in cases of great irritability, attended with vomiting, gives prompt relief.

Poppy Fomentation.

Take white poppy heads; simmer them in equal parts of vinegar and water. This is an excellent anodyne application in painful affections.

GARGLES.

Gargles, in many complaints, are useful, particularly in quinzy, apthea, or sore throat, fevers, &c. By this class of medicines, we understand certain infusions, or liquids, suitable for washing the mouth, which, by their stimulating or detergent properties, become very efficacious. Adults can gargle their throat, or mouth, with little difficulty; but children require an assistant to apply them, which is best done by tying a piece of linen to a probe, or stick, dipping it in the liquid and applying it often. They should not be very stimulating, except in severe cases.

30. *Astringent Gargle.*

Take of bayberry bark, hemlock bark, white pond lily root, red raspberry leaves, witch hazel bark, or leaves, blue scabish, of each, one ounce; boil, make a strong decoction, and sweeten with honey.

This gargle is used with great success in almost all cases of sore mouth and throat. A little cayenne pepper may be added with advantage. This preparation is also used extensively as a wash in ulcers, canker, sores, &c.

31. *Stimulating Gargle.*

Take of sumach berries one ounce, golden seal one ounce, cayenne pepper half an ounce, water one pint; boil, and add one drachm of alum.

Used in sore throat generally. Slippery elm may be added.

TINCTURES.

Tinctures are certain active ingredients, principally vegetable substances, which are imparted to spirits, alcohol, or wine. They are excellent for administering a great variety of medicinal agents, but in some cases there may be an objection to them in consequence of the spirits they contain. They yield their virtues more readily by the addition of heat.

32. *Compound Tincture of Myrrh, or Vegetable Elixir.*

Take of gum myrrh, pulverized, half pound, cayenne pepper two ounces, whiskey, or gin, one gallon; put the whole into a stone jug; set it into a kettle of water and boil it fifteen or twenty minutes, leaving the cork out.

This elixir, or tincture, in point of utility, is surpassed by none, either for internal or external application. In cases of pain in the stomach or bowels, recent diarrhœa, cramp, and for pain in the limbs and head, it is applied with great advantage; and finally, there is scarcely a case of disease where it may not be profitably employed, except in cases of acute inflammation internally—in which case it should be used sparingly. It powerfully resists mortification. It may be prepared in the same manner with alcohol, spirits of wine, or fourth proof brandy, which makes it more powerful, and is considered by some practitioners preferable to common spirits.—This preparation is called *Hot Drops, No.* 6, &c. To one ounce of the drops, add one ounce spirits turpentine, and it forms a valuable itch-ointment.

33. *Tincture of Lobelia.*

Take of lobelia herb one ounce, valerian one ounce,

spirits one quart; shake it occasionally for several days; then strain and keep it corked.

The tincture of lobelia forms an excellent emetic for children, in doses of a teaspoonful. It is used with almost certain success in asthma, croup, inflammation of the lungs, &c.

34. *Sudorific Tincture.*

Take of ipecac one ounce, saffron one ounce, camphor one ounce, Virginia snake root one ounce, valerian one ounce, gin, or rum, one quart; let it stand two weeks and filter.

Dose.—A teaspoonful, in a cup of catnip or saxifrage tea, every hour, until it produces perspiration.

Use.—This preparation is useful in fevers, inflammations, &c. to produce perspiration.

INFUSIONS.

Infusion is a very good method of administering the virtues of various medicinal agents. A two-fold advantage is derived from infusion:—*First*, the medicinal properties of the article made use of. *Second*, the heat and diluent properties of the water; but no medicine should be administered of higher temperature than blood heat.

Compound infusion of Senna.

Take of Senna one ounce, manna one ounce, fennel seed one ounce, boiling water one pint; simmer to half pint, and sweeten with molasses.

Dose.—A wine-glass full every hour until it operates.

Use.—A cooling purgative in fevers, and inflammatory diseases generally.

35. *Mucilaginous infusion.*

Take of slippery elm bark one ounce, flax-seed one ounce, boiling water three pints. This forms a useful demulcent drink in gonorrhœa, disuary, cough, catarrh, &c.

INJECTIONS, OR CLYSTERS.

Injections, or clysters, are certain liquid preparations thrown into the rectum by mechanical means. Their operation, or effect, depends on the ingredient used.—Some are emollient, others are stimulant, anodyne, purgative, antispasmodic, &c. A large syringe should be used for adults, and a small one for children; which renders it easy to perform this simple and yet valuable operation efficiently. Few are aware of the great benefit which may be received from their use. They often prove a sovereign remedy for diseases which nothing else will relieve, and a simple clyster can seldom do any injury. Hence every family should possess a syringe, and a knowledge of its use.

Sometimes the stomach is in such a situation that medicine cannot be given to act upon the bowels, and it never can be with that certainty of success in any other form, that it can in clysters. They are used with great benefit in cholic, dysentery, piles, cholera morbus, costiveness, stranguary, gravel, diabetes, falling of the rectum, fluor albus, flowings, stoppage of the courses, pain in the back, and all hysterical affections. When there is a tendency to delirium, or inflammation of the head, the emetic should first be given to clear the stomach.

36. *Stimulating Injection.*

Take of bayberry bark two ounces, hemlock bark two ounces, white pond lily root two ounces, witch hazel leaves one ounce, raspberry leaves one ounce; make a strong infusion; to half a pint, add half a gill of molasses, one teaspoonful lobelia, and one teaspoonful cayenne pepper. Inject half a pint; if this dose does not produce a movement in the bowels, from half to a teaspoonful of spirits turpentine may be added.

This preparation is very active, and often gives relief when all other means fail. It is used in billious cholic, stranguary, gravel, and obstinate costiveness; and in most cases where the emetic is given, it may be given with advantage.

37. *Emollient Injection*

Take of olive oil two ounces, mucilage of slippery elm four ounces, molasses two ounces, sweet milk half a pint, saleratus one scruple, or a piece the size of a small walnut.

This is a preparation of much value. It is used in dysentery, diarrhœa, and in all cases where stimulating injections are not proper.

38. *Common Injection.*

Take of common yest one gill, sweet milk two gills, molasses one gill. This preparation is useful in any case where an injection is required, but is not equal to either of the above.

LINAMENTS.

Linaments are preparations employed in frictions or embrocations of the skin; they are usually composed of oily spiritous and gummy or suponaceous substances, as some of the essential oils, alcohol, soap, camphor, &c. They are used externally for rheumatism, quinzy, and other painful affections. The principal benefit is derived from their counter irritant effects; they may also give elasticity and strength to the muscles.

39. *Compound Linament.*

Take of neats foot oil one pint, olive oil one gill, brandy two gills, mix and simmer slowly until the water is evaporated; then let it cool to blood heat; add spirits turpentine half a gill.

Use.—This linament is useful for swellings of various kinds, where suppuration has not commenced; and for sprains, bruises, contusions, shrunk sinews, stiff joints, rheumatism, &c. it is probably not surpassed by any similar preparation. Half an ounce of cayenne pepper, and half an ounce of lobelia, may be added before it is simmered, which renders it more stimulating, and in some cases preferable.

40. *Aromatic Linament.*

Take of oil of sassafras one ounce, camphor one ounce, spirits of hartshorne one ounce, castile soap one ounce, oil of hemlock one ounce, alcohol four ounces.

Use.—This is an excellent application in diseases of the throat and tonsils, and for rheumatism, &c.

41. *Rheumatic Linament.*

Take of alcohol two quarts, castile soap one ounce, sassafras oil one ounce, spearmint oil one ounce, oil origanum one ounce, oil of amber one ounce; put the whole into a stone jug, keep it warm four or five days, and shake it often.

Use.—This linament is useful in rheumatism, sprains, and other painful affections.

42. *Discutient Linament.*

Take of alcohol or brandy two gills, oil of spike one gill; British oil one ounce, camphor one ounce, salt-petre one ounce. This linament is used for rheumatism, sprains, &c. &c. It is powerful, and should be used sparingly.

POULTICES.

Poultices, or cataplasms, are external applications, of a soft or pulpy consistence, and somewhat tenacious. They are of various kinds, some being designed for discutients, others to produce suppuration; some are refrigerent, or cooling, other stimulating, and others again emollient. In general, poultices should be applied warm, and not suffered to get dry.

42. *Compound Yest Poultice.*

Take of black birch bark and blue or water beecn,

equal parts; make a strong decoction; to two quarts of the decoction add four ounces white hellebore; boil fifteen minutes, then strain and add slippery elm bark pulverized, and indian meal, sufficient to form a poultice; then add of good yest one gill, sal-eratus one drachm, and lobelia half an ounce.

Use.—This poultice is excelled by none of which we have any knowledge, for local inflamations of a painful nature; it may be applied to the back in inflammations of the kidneys, and the side in pleurisy, &c.

44. *Alkaline Poultice.*

Take of common ley, blood warm and rather weak, and stir in slippery elm bark sufficient to form a poultice.

This poultice is useful in inflamation of the breast, felons, white swelling, inflamed wounds, &c.

45. *Mustard Poultice.*

Take of mustard seed pulverized four ounces, soft bread or Indian meal six ounces, cayenne pepper half an ounce, and vinegar of the best quality sufficient to form a poultice.

Use.—This poultice may be applied to the soles of the feet and other parts, in fevers, inflammations, and rheumatisms.

46. *Elm Poultice.*

Take milk and water, boiling hot, and stir in elm bark. This poultice is used in all cases of inflammation, and sores of every description.

47. *Detergent Poultice.*

Take of bayberry bark, hemlock bark, white lily root, raspberry leaves, witch hazel leaves, marsh rosemary, and blue scabish, equal parts, or any part, if the whole cannot be obtained; make a strong decoction; then add common crackers, pulverized, and slippery elm bark, equal parts, and ginger one spoonful. This poultice is particularly useful in the treatment of scrofulous, canker, and other sores generally; for old fever sores it possesses superior efficacy.

CAUSTICS.

Caustics and escharotics are those substances which, when applied to fungus-flesh, or the skin, decompose and remove it.

48. *Alkaline Caustic.*

Take walnut or white-oak ashes; leach them; boil the ley until it forms a pot-ash; then dry it gradually, and pulverize; keep it from the air.

Use.—This caustic may be applied to fungus, or proud-flesh; and, frequently applied, excites discharge from indolent swellings, and is in some cases preferable to opening by incision.

49. *Vegetable Caustic.*

Take of dragon's tooth and blood root, pulverized, equal parts. This caustic is useful in the treatment of ulcers, fever-sores, &c.

50 *Mineral Caustic.*

Take of copperas and alum, equal parts; submit it to a moderate heat until it is decomposed, or burnt; then pulverize and mix; keep it in glass vessels from the air.

Useful to remove fungus, or dead flesh.

SALVES.

Salves are medicines of proper consistence for spreading on linen, or muslin, designed for external application. They are formed by uniting wax, resin, or oil, with some remedial agents, either vegetable or some of the metalic oxides—such as red lead, &c. They are used for ulcers, wounds, &c.

51. *Black Salve.*

Take of linseed oil one pint, neat's-foot oil one pint, bee's wax four ounces, rosin twelve ounces, gum arabic four ounces, gum camphor one ounce, rum one gill; melt these together; then add, of red lead one pound, white lead one pound; the leads should be finely pulverized and sifted; stir until cool.

This salve is used in fever-sores, scurvy, sores, &c.

52. *Vegetable Salve.*

Take of bayberry tallow eight ounces, turpentine eight ounces, mutton tallow two ounces, or olive oil one ounce; melt together, and stir till cool. This salve is valuable for most kinds of common sores.

53. *Green Salve.*

Take of rosin one pound, bee's wax eight ounces, turpentine eight ounces, balsam fir eight ounces, sweet oil two ounces, verdigris the sixteenth of an ounce; melt and stir until cool.

This is, of all salves, the most valuable for old ulcers, fever sores, scurvy sores, &c. and may be used for cuts, burns, and sores generally. It may be used without the verdigris in fresh wounds, and lobelia seed may be added for bad ulcers.

OINTMENTS.

Ointments are a class of medicines which contain the properties of certain vegetables, designed for external application. Their consistence is softer than salves, or plaster, but the heat of the body is sufficient to melt them. Lard and butter, or oil, are principally used in making.

According to the direction given in the dispensatories, the properties of vegetables are not communicated to either of these substances through the medium of water alone, particularly if they are dry; but by simmering them in spirits, the desired object may be obtained.

54. *Lettuce Ointment.*

Take of the extract of wild lettuce one pint, hog's lard one pound, turpentine eight ounces; simmer very slow, and stir until thoroughly incorporated; then stir until cool.

This ointment is used for excoriation of the nipples, for which it is very valuable, and should be applied immediately after the child nurses; it will also benefit the child's mouth, if sore; it is also useful for sore lips, cracked hands, &c.

55. *Little's Burn Ointment.*

Take of lard one pound, sulphur one ounce, tar two ounces, verdigris one drachm; melt and stir until cool. This ointment is useful for burns, scald-head, itch, herpetic affections, &c.

56. *Green Ointment.*

Take tanzy, worm-wood, hoarhound, catnip, and hops, of each one ounce; bruise; put it in a brass or tin vessel; add spirits two quarts, melted lard one pound; let it digest one week; then boil and strain it; then boil to the consistence of tar. This ointment is cooling, relaxing, emollient, and resolvent; useful in sprains, swellings, dislocations, and contracted sinews.

57. *Tetter Ointment.*

Take of turpentine eight ounces, fresh butter eight ounces, olive oil one ounce, bee's wax two ounces, Indian turnip, fresh plant, one ounce, white lily one ounce, common plaintain one ounce; put the whole into an earthen vessel, cover close, and simmer very slow two hours; then strain; and when nearly cold, add two drachms yellow ochre.

This ointment is very useful in tetters, salt-rheum, herpetic affections, &c.

58. *Itch Ointment.*

Take of lard one pound, Venice turpentine one ounce, sulphur one ounce; melt them together, and stir until cold.

This ointment cures the itch in a short time, and with little trouble.

59. *Ophthalmic Ointment.*

Take of garden celendine four ounces, fresh butter eight ounces; put them into an earthern vessel; simmer slow twelve hours; be careful not to burn or crisp the herb. This ointment is emollient, and cooling; useful for removing film from the eyes, and for most cases of sore eyes where the inflammation is not high. It is also valuable for the cure of piles.

60. *Compound Ointment.*

Take of lettuce ointment one ounce, cancer plaster, No. 65, one ounce, mutton tallow four ounces; melt the tallow; then add the other ingredients, and stir until cool. This ointment is useful in the treatment of cancers, scrofulous, and herpetic affections; to be applied after poultices, caustics, &c.

61. *Elder Ointment.*

Take of the bark of sweet elder, two ounces, the bark of the root of black-berry brier two ounces, sweet cream one pint; simmer in a tin or pewter vessel six hours, then strain.

This ointment is very useful for external poisons—by ivy, sumach, and other poison vegetables. The inflammation should be first removed by applying the detergent, or other poultices.

62. *Emollient Ointment.*

Take of the root of bitter-sweet one pound, camomile eight ounces, worm-wood eight ounces, yellow dock leaves four ounces, cayenne pepper one ounce, neat's-foot oil one gallon, cogniac brandy one quart; simmer the whole in a moderate heat twelve hours; then strain, and add two ounces spirits turpentine to each pound of the ointment. This ointment is used for callouses, hard swellings, shrunk sinews, stiff joints, corns, &c.

PLASTERS.

Plasters have generally for their base, resin, wax, gum, or pitch, combined with extracts, oils, oxides, &c. and are designed to adhere to the parts without melting.

63. *Strengthening Plaster.*

Take of rosin one pound, turpentine four ounces, bole Armenian one ounce, dregs of vegetable elixir two ounces, mutton tallow two ounces; melt the whole; and when thoroughly incorporated, pour into cold water, and work it with your hands until it will swim on the surface.

This is a valuable plaster for removing pain, and strengthening the parts to which it is applied. It may be applied to the loins, side, or any other part.

64. *Black Plaster.*

Take of the extract of white oak bark eight ounces, extract of the bark and buds of the balm of Gilead eight ounces, rosin eight ounces, turpentine four ounces, mutton tallow two ounces; melt and work in water.

This plaster is applied, with extraordinary benefit, to weak and painful joints, occasioned by dislocation, rheumatism, strains, &c. and is very useful for pain in the side and back.

65. *Cancer Plaster.*

Take red field clover heads, when in blossom; put into a brass kettle; add water; boil and strain, and then boil until it forms an extract; be careful not to burn it.

Use.—This forms an excellent plaster for cancers, scrofulous, and herpetic affections.

66. *Ferris' Plaster.*

Take white oak bark, cut fine; cover it with urine; let it digest for three days; then boil, strain, and boil to the consistence of tar. To five pounds of the extract, add honey one pound, turpentine one pound; add two drachms of white vitriol, when designed to act as an escharotic, or caustic.

Use.—This forms a valuable plaster for cancers, ulcers, and white swellings in a state of ulceration, and for removing fungus flesh. It excites but little pain or inflammation.

67. *Sorrel Plaster.*

Take wood-sorrel; bruise, and press out the juice; put it in a pewter or bright tin plate; expose it to the heat and light of the sun; dry it to the consistence of tar; then add one drachm of alum to one ounce of the plaster; keep it in a glass vessel from the air.

This plaster is probably not surpassed by any other for the treatment of some species of cancers.

68. *Adhesive Plaster.*

Take of white rosin three pounds, bee's wax four ounces, Burgundy pitch two pounds, mutton tallow four ounces; melt these together; then add olive oil half an ounce, camphor half an ounce, West India rum one gill, sassafras oil half an ounce. When the whole is thoroughly incorporated, pour into cold water, and work with the hands until cold.

This is a valuable plaster for dressing wounds and ulcers, and a strengthening plaster. It is perhaps equal to any of its character that has been used.

PILLS.

Pills are small, round substances, composed of vegetable medicines; rather hard. The unpleasant taste, or smell, of the medicine is thereby concealed from the palate, and rendered less offensive. They are longer in digesting, and consequently have a more general effect upon the stomach and bowels.

69. *Cathartic Pill.*

Take of lobelia herb, pulverized, one ounce; add water one gill; boil it until the water is evaporated; then add mandrake root one ounce, extract of butternut bark one ounce, cayenne pepper one ounce; the extract of lobelia may be used instead of the powder, half an ounce; it is perhaps preferable to the powder.

Use.—These pills form a valuable cathartic for cleansing the stomach and bowels; they are very active and stimulating. Dose—from two to four.

70. *Billious Pill.*

Take of gamboge one ounce, aloes three ounces, rheubarb three ounces, castile soap two ounces, jalap two ounces, lobelia one ounce, cayenne pepper two ounces, molasses sufficient to prepare it for rolling.

Dose—from two to six. These pills are useful in billious and dyspeptic habits, and in most cases where a mild cathartic is required.

71. *White Pill.*

Take of spikenard one ounce, slippery elm bark one ounce, comfrey one ounce, cayenne pepper half an ounce, lobelia one fourth of an ounce, molasses one gill; roll them in pulverized loaf sugar.

Useful for weak stomach, and general debility.

72. *Restorative Pill.*

Take of golden seal four ounces, valerian four ounces, bitter root four ounces, lobelia one ounce, cayenne pepper one ounce, tumeric balsam, or gum, one ounce, extract of butternut, or peach tree bark, sufficient to prepare it for rolling.

These pills are an excellent restorative in dyspepsia, female complaints, &c.

BITTERS.

By this class of medicines, we understand certain liquids, as wine or spirits, impregnated with those vegetables which contain the greatest quantity of the bitter principle. They are used to impart tone and energy to the stomach.

73. *Stomach Bitters.*

Take of balmony two ounces, poplar bark two ounces, bayberry bark two ounces, boneset two ounces, bugle one ounce; pulverize; add boiling water one gallon, spirits two quarts.

These bitters are very valuable in billious habits, dyspepsia, and loss of appetite; in the last of which they are superior to all others.

Dose.—A wine-glass full two or three times a day.

74. *Wine Bitters.*

Take of golden seal two ounces, white-wood bark two ounces, bitter-sweet two ounces, cayenne pepper one ounce, wine two gallons.

Dose.—From a spoonful to a wine-glass full.

These bitters are a very good tonic for dyspepsia, debility, &c.

75. *Compound Bitters.*

Take of wild cherry bark one pound, turmeric bark two pounds, prickly ash bark one pound, seneca snake root one pound, tanzy four ounces, socotrine aloes three ounces; pulverize; to four ounces of the mixture add three pints boiling water, and two quarts of gin.

These bitters are valuable for dyspepsia, obstructed menses, and other diseases where tonics are required.

76. *Spice Bitters.*

Take of allspice two ounces, prickly ash berries, or bark, two ounces, golden seal two ounces, poplar bark two ounces, gentian, or bitter-root, two ounces, boneset two ounces, spirits one gallon, or wine two gallons.

These bitters form a valuable tonic for general debility, female weaknesses, relaxed habits, low state of the blood, &c.

78. Eye Waters.

Eye waters are prepared from vegetable or mineral substances, added to spirits, or water, and applied in form of a wash. They should be applied very weak, and the strength increased gradually.

79. *Compound Eye Water.*

Take of bayberry bark, raspberry leaves, witch hazel leaves, and lobelia herb, equal parts; make a strong infusion; to one gill, add one teaspoonful of vegetable elixir.

This eye water is used in all cases of sore or weak eyes.

80. *Vegetable Eye Water.*

Take red willow; make a strong infusion; a little brandy may be added.

This forms a valuable application for the eyes, particularly in cases of inflammation.

81. *Mucilaginous Eye Water.*

Take the pith of sassafras shrubs; infuse in cold water; add rose-water. This forms a cooling wash for the eyes.

82. *Welch Medicamentum.*

Take of aloes four ounces, rheubarb four ounces, ginger one pound, brown sugar two pounds, spirits one gallon, essence of peppermint one ounce; put the whole together; shake it occasionally for two or three days.

Dose.—A tablespoonful for an adult; for a child a teaspoonful.

Use.—This very valuable compound is used in costiveness, indigestion, loss of appetite, billious complaints, worms in children, &c.

83. *Mustard Linament.*

Take of mustard seed, pulverized, two ounces, camphor one ounce, rattlesnake's oil one ounce, opium half an ounce, alcohol two quarts; put the whole into a glass bottle; keep warm.

This linament is used for broken limbs that remain swelled, or painful, after the bone is healed, and is said to be very useful.

84. *Opodeldoc.*

Take of alcohol one quart, Windsor soap eight ounces, camphor two ounces, oil of rosemary one eighth of an ounce; any other aromatic oil may be used.

85. *Welch Elixir.*

Take of aloes four ounces, saffron one ounce, Venice treacle one ounce, white agerate one ounce, wormwood essence one fourth of an ounce, essence of aniseseed two ounces, brandy two quarts; put the whole into a glass bottle; cover with parchment; make holes in the parchment with a pin; shake it daily for one week; then cork it tight, and keep for use.

This is said to be a very useful family medicine for indigestion, costiveness, &c. and is a good tonic.

86. *Little's Mineral Water.*

Take of white vitriol one drachm, crocus martus two drachms, water one quart; shake it daily one week.

This forms an excellent wash for fever-sores, &c. and a very valuable eye water. It will often cure sooner than any other preparation.

87. *Scorbutic Wash.*

Take spirits one pint, blood root one ounce, dragon's claw one ounce, lobelia one ounce; mix and shake well together.

This forms a valuable application for affections of the skin, particularly of the face; it will remove pimples and other eruptions in a short time.

88. *Neutralizing Cordial.*

Take of rheubarb two ounces, saleratus one ounce, peppermint plant one ounce, hot water one quart, loaf sugar eight ounces.

This mixture is useful in dysentery, cholera morbus, diarrhœa, &c.

89. *Compound Tincture of Lobelia.*

Take of lobelia seed, pulverized, two ounces, cayenne pepper two ounces, valerian half an ounce, vegetable elixir one pint; put the whole into a bottle, and shake it occasionally.

Use.—This preparation is used for all sudden attacks of diseases, such as spasms, fits, lock-jaw, and poisons; and all cases when a quick and active emetic is required. This is called third preparation, &c.

90. *Cream Cordial.*

Take of sweet cream one gill, water half a gill, vegetable elixir half a gill, Bateman's drops one fourth of a gill, tincture of lobelia one tablespoonful, loaf sugar four ounces.

This cordial is a valuable preparation for patients recovering from severe attacks of disease. It is an excellent tonic and restorative.

91. *Sudorific Powders.*

Take of May-weed, meadow-saxifrage, catnip, and white snake root, equal parts; pulverize.

This powder is very useful for producing perspiration, or sweating. It may be given in the powder or infusion.

92. *Emetic Pill.*

Take of lobelia seed, pulverized, one ounce, cayenne pepper one ounce, extract of butternut two ounces; roll them in flour.

These pills are valuable in chronic diseases, such as affections of the liver, spleen, &c. The extract of lobelia may be used instead of the seed.

Dose.—From one to three on going to bed, every night.

93. *Detergent Powder.*

Take of bayberry bark, hemlock bark, white lily root, witch hazel bark, or leaves, red raspberry leaves, and blue scabish, equal parts; pulverize.

This powder is useful to remove canker, and may be used for that in its varied forms. The infusion forms an excellent wash for sores of every kind, sore mouth, &c.

94. *Neutralizing Mixture.*

Take of rheubarb, pulverized, one ounce, soda one ounce; mix thoroughly.

Use.—These powders possess surprising power in neutralizing the acidity of the stomach.

Dose.—From one fourth to a teaspoonful.

THE VAPOR BATH.

The use of the vapor or steam bath, is very important in many cases for removing disease, if properly applied. In acute, inflammatory diseases, such as pleurisy, rheumatism, and fevers, and also in cases of suspended animation from drowning, or other causes, it is of the utmost importance. It is peculiarly adapted to imparting heat to the system, and promoting and establishing a free perspiration, which is one of the most important evacuations of the system. The following is the most convenient method of applying the vapor, or steam:—Make a frame, circular or otherwise, so constructed that it may be raised or lowered at pleasure; cover it with canvass; let the patient stand or sit within this enclosure; close the canvass about the neck, and introduce the steam by means of a tin pipe, from a boiler, placed over a stove or fire-place, in such a manner that it does not strike directly on the patient. Or the following plan answers very well:—Cover the patient with a blanket, except the head; let him sit in a chair, or stand up; place a vessel, containing boiling water, at his feet; put a stone into the water of ten or fifteen pounds weight, previously heated; then enclose the vessel with the blanket which covers the patient, and change the stones occasionally, as they cool. If the patient is unable to sit up, the steam may be applied in bed, by raising the clothes, and supporting them by means of sticks, or semi-circular hoops; then introduce the steam as above. It is important that the steam should strike every part of the body. The steam should be continued, according to the strength of the patient, from fifteen to thirty minutes, or until a free perspiration is produced. Great care should be taken not to raise the external heat too fast in proportion to the internal heat. To prevent this, give freely of the alterative powders, vegetable elixir, cayenne pepper, or other suitable stimulants. The patient should always be supplied with drink of a sudorific nature, such as the infusion of white snake root, meadow saxifrage, boneset, or May-weed. The heat should not be raised so high as to be oppressive or suffocating to the patient, as it is never necessary nor beneficial. After sweating sufficiently, the patient should be washed with the vegetable elixir, vinegar, or water, rather cool, to prevent the morbid matter, which is thrown off by perspiration, from being re-absorbed by the pores of the skin. Weak ley is recommended as a wash, and frequently used to advantage, as it effectually removes those oily or glutinous substances which collect on the skin.

THE DRY VAPOR BATH.

This vapor is applied by shielding the patient from the air, as directed under the head of vapor or steam bath; then place a vessel containing half a pint of spirits within the enclosure, set it on fire, and let the patient be exposed to the action of the vapor until the spirits are evaporated, or until a free perspiration is produced.—This bath may be substituted for the steam vapor in most cases, except in inflammatory diseases.

PART IV.

PHYSIOLOGY,

OR THE DESCRIPTION AND TREATMENT OF DISEASES.

A SHORT DESCRIPTION OF THE NATURE AND CAUSES OF FEVER.

Fever is an increased action of the heart and arteries, to expel from the system irritating or morbific matter.—It is salutary in its nature, being the means used to throw off something that offends or oppresses her. It is often fatal, but this is rather to be attributed to the fault of the constitution than to the disease itself, or rather to the want of proper medicines to assist nature in her work.—As much controversy and speculation as there is respecting the pathology or nature of fever, we think there is no complaint more simple or easily understood, as regards causes, symptoms, and treatment.

We may consider fever a unit; that the various phenomena of the complaint depend not on any specific difference in the many types of fever, but consist rather in the various exciting causes, habit, temperament, &c.

The remote causes of fever are very numerous and various. High atmospheric temperature may be mentioned as a cause; but cold, united with moisture, is the most fruitful source of disease. The deleterious effluvia arising from the decomposition of vegetable substances; from persons in a state of disease; from putrid animal substances; are among the remote, but not least exciting causes, of fever. Daily experience confirms the fact, that in the neighborhood of marshes, and all such places, where vegetable and animal putrefaction takes place to any extent, pestilential and other diseases of various grades and violence, prevail. Epidemics, attended with carbuncles and buboes, which are denominated, in conjunction with other ordinary symptoms, of what is called jail and hospital fever, the characteristics of the plague, down to the mildest intermittents, have appeared and raged with extraordinary violence, occasioned by the exhalations from putrifying animal and vegetable substances.

Among the intermediate or less remote causes of fever, is a morbid state of the stomach, arising from vitiated bile, which is almost universally the case, (to a greater or less extent,) from canker seated in the stomach and bowels. Another very important intermediate cause, is obstruction in the capillary vessels, or pores.

The proximate or immediate cause of fever, is a retention of acrid, stimulating, or morbific matter or humors, which, instead of being carried off by the out-lets or excretions of the system, enter the circulation, and stimulate the heart and arteries to undue and increased action, to overcome the obstruction of the capillary vessels, and expel such morbific matter. The seat of fever, then, is in the blood vessels, or the vascular system. It is well known that a greater or less degree of fever, invariably follows a sudden check of perspiration. Hence it is evident that the exciting cause must be in the blood, and arise from an excess of stimulating or corroding matter, which may be generated in the system without any external exciting cause; or by means of the action of deleterious effluvia upon the lungs and stomach, and thus communicating with the blood.

This fact is demonstrated by the phenomena of eruptive diseases, as small pox, measles, &c. This infection, or contagion, is taken into the blood through the medium of the lungs, and as soon as it becomes sufficiently impregnated with the specific humor, or virus, a preternatural action of the blood vessels immediately takes place. Nature is aroused, and makes a powerful effort, or struggle, to expel the poison from the system. As soon as she accomplishes this object, the exciting cause or agent in these eruptive complaints is thrown copiously to the surface, and appears in the form of vesicles or eruptions; and when they are thus expelled, the fever immediately subsides, but will re-appear if from debility or other causes, the poison or humor is absorbed. It is the case also in hectic fever, as almost every one knows, matter from the lungs, or an ulcer, is taken into the circulation, and causes fever. It is also proved from the termination of fevers by sweating. These facts reduce it to a mathematical demonstration, and render the subject so simple and plain, that it is really a matter of profound astonishment that any one, the least acquainted with fevers, should be ignorant of their cause and cure. These facts are abundantly supported by the most eminent writers of the old school, both ancient and modern.

To sum in a word, we may say, that all febrile diseases, or fevers, are caused by cold and obstructions in the system.

SYMPTOMS.

The first characteristic symptoms of fever, are rigor, or chills, succeeded by a preternatural degree of heat.—Sometimes the chill is very severe; at others, very light; but fever is almost invariably ushered in by this symptom. The patient complains of great coldness; he shakes and trembles; the skin is pale, rough, and shrunken; and sometimes there is a sensation like cold water running down the back. After a while the chilliness subsides, and flushing and heat prevail, with a return of the color of the skin. The eyes become red, and the patient now complains of heat. The continuance of the cold stage is very uncertain. Sometimes it lasts an hour; at others, it continues several days, with alternate flushings of heat.

Another symptom of fever, is an increased frequency of the pulse. It usually becomes more frequent, full, and hard, showing clearly the increased action of the heart and arteries, which, however, are modified or altered by various incidental circumstances; by some of the passions; by diet, exercise, air, medicine, &c. Debility is an invariable attendant of fever. There is a sense of languor and fatigue which is generally increased by any exertion.

Pain is usually felt in the head, along the spine, (or back bone,) and in the joints.

All the secretions and excretions are deranged on or before the accession of fevers. The tongue appears coated with a foul substance, and this serves as an index to point out the accumulation of billious matter in the stomach. There is usually loss of appetite, nausea, and vomiting. The mouth is dry and clammy, from an obstruction of the salivary glands; the skin dry and parched, from diminished perspiration; the urine is scanty and high colored, and there is generally a constipation of the bowels. In a word, all the functions of the system are impaired.

It is therefore exceedingly important, in a practical point of view, to bear in mind the method invariably adopted by nature to cure a fever, which is the restoration of the secretions; and in most cases it is by sweat, or perspiration. Without this knowledge, there would be a fatal error in practice; but when we are well apprised of this fact, we shall at once know what indications to fulfil, or in other words, what course of treatment to pursue. The whole business of art, therefore, is to assist nature in these two efforts of excretion and secretion of the morbific matter.

To fulfil these indications, particular attention to the different organs of the system, such as the stomach, bowels, and kidneys, and also the capillary system, or pores of the skin, is called for.

THE STOMACH.

When we reflect upon the extensive influence of the stomach over the system, and particularly the skin, we shall be able more readily to appreciate the utility of emetics in febrile diseases. It is by reason of this intimate relation and connexion between the stomach and every part of the system, that the administration of an emetic proves so very effectual. It not only cleanses the stomach of any billious, feculent, irritating or morbific matter, but it also proves eminently beneficial by the general relaxation which it produces, and which extends to the skin and produces perspiration. They may as a general rule, be given in all cases where there is no peculiarity of the constitution to forbid. Even when the stomach appears to be thoroughly cleansed, they may be advantageously given, in consequence of the shock and stimulating effect given to the stomach, liver, and the whole system. Hence appears the impropriety of giving powerful cathartics, as they carry the offending matter through the bowels, which of course absorb a greater or less quantity of it, and are consequently deranged.

THE BOWELS.

The intimate relation which exists between the alimentary canal, or bowels, and the skin, and other parts of the animal economy, points out the necessity of promoting in them a healthy action. For this purpose, clysters, or injections, are preferable to any other class of medicines. The preternatural excitement of the blood vessels, is sensibly diminished by their exhibition. This effect is produced by stimulating the exhalent vessels of the mucous membrane of the intestines, causing them to pour out copious effusions of morbific matter from the blood, or circulating mass. Their importance must be seen in a striking point of view, when the length of the intestines is considered, (which is about thirty feet,) and also their office. There are an immense number of vessels opening into them through their whole extent, and from which there is poured out a vast quantity of feculant matter; and when there is a preternatural stimulus given to the intestines, there is a sympathetic affection of the whole system, and there is also always more or less canker in the bowels, which is a fruitful source of disease. This cannot be removed as readily by any other means as by suitable clysters, or injections. Mild cathartics, however, in moderate doses, are useful after the stomach has been cleansed by emetics; and they may be given in larger doses when any peculiarity in the constitution of the patient forbids giving emetics.

THE PORES, OR CAPILLARY SYSTEM.

It appears that febrile diseases, in their very nature and essence, consist in a derangement of the skin, or capillary system, and that no means will subdue a fever until this function is restored. We must be convinced of the necessity of this, from the extensive surface of the skin, its connection with the stomach and sanguiferous system, and its important office in casting off superfluous and noxious matter. It is calculated that from one half to two thirds of what is taken into the system, is evaporated by sensible or insensible perspiration. Hence it will be seen what mischief must follow from a retention of this perishable matter, and what benefit will follow by restoring this secretion. For this purpore, the vapor bath, accompanied with stimulating and sudorific, or sweating medicines, are the best means that can be employed. It is also frequently beneficial to bathe the whole surface with weak ley-water, which removes the glutinous substance that adheres to it.

THE KIDNEYS.

When the kidneys cease to perform their offices, or do it imperfectly, the urine becomes scanty, or much diminished. This fluid is retained, carried into the circulation, and must prove a source of irritation; and hence the necessity of restoring the secretion of it.

Diuretic medicines, therefore, or such as promote a discharge of urine, and allay the irritation of these organs, must be administered. For this purpose, the effusion of queen of the meadow, juniper, and dwarf elder, or spearmint, may be given.

THE LUNGS.

The lungs are an organ to which particular attention should be paid. They are the main-spring of the system their office being to supply it with the vital principle.—If this is withheld, or they absorb impure air, the fever is exasperated. It is therefore necessary to place the patient in a well ventilated room, where the air has a free circulation, yet it should not be allowed to strike immediately upon the patient.

THE FEET.

It is generally known that fevers are frequently occasioned by the application of cold to the feet, which drives the blood from the extremities, and throws it upon some organ, or retains such agents as ought to be thrown off; in consequence of which, fever takes place. Now it must be evident that there is no better method of preventing these consequences than by bathing the feet in warm water, or applying steam to them, thereby recalling the blood to the surface and extremeties.

Draughts applied to the feet are very important in febrile diseases generally.

A general course of treatment for febrile diseases.

As a general rule, the following course may be adopted in all febrile diseases, or cases of fever, in its various types, and will fully answer all the forementioned indications:—Give first suitable stimulants to raise the internal heat, as the alterative powders, cayenne pepper, vegetable elixir, &c. Then apply the vapor or steam bath as before described, until a brisk perspiration is produced; then give the stimulating injection No 36; and then emetic No. 3; and repeat it until it operates thoroughly. Then when the patient is a little rested, apply the vapor bath again; wash the whole surface, and change the under-clothes; then give a moderate cathartic, merely sufficient to cause a slight action of the bowels. Then give the alterative powders, or other stimulants, once in two or three hours, to keep up the internal heat; and repeat the above course at intervals of from twelve to forty-eight hours, until relief is obtained.—

When the fever is allayed, give suitable medicines to restore the digestive powers and strengthen the system. For this purpose, give the tonic syrup, No. 9, antidysenteric cordial, No. 16, the stomach bitters, No. 73, or wine bitters, No. 78, &c. according to the situation of the patient. Attention should be paid to particular symptoms, such as soreness of the throat, pain in the head, and other parts, from congestion, or an unusual quantity of blood thrown upon some other organ. If there is pain in the head, cold applications should be used. For this purpose, the lobelia fomentation, No. 26, is superior to all others. Salt and vinegar may be used, and bitter fomentations.

QUIETUDE OF BODY AND MIND.

It is of the utmost importance to keep the patient as quiet as possible, and prevent all unnecessary exertion. The mind should also be kept perfectly at ease, and all causes of alarm or excitement carefully avoided.

DRINKS.

Drink should always be given freely in fevers, as they furnish a suitable vehicle for carrying off the morbid matter by perspiration and urine, and should therefore be of a sudorific, diaphoretic, or diuretic kind; but if the patient desire it, he may take water, rather cool, with the addition of a little burning charcoal, a roasted apple while hot, or a little lemonade. But no cool drink should be given during the operation of the emetic, or immediately after.

REGIMEN.

The dictates of nature should be followed in a measure, as regards regimen, or food, in fevers. Although the patient has the greatest inclination for drink, yet he has seldom any appetite for solid food. Hence the absurdity of urging him to take victuals, or much solid food in fever, as it is injurious. It oppresses the stomach, and instead of nourishing the patient, serves only to increase the disease. The food that is taken, should be very light, vegetable, and easy of digestion, consisting chiefly of panada, thin gruel, or roasted apples; and as the digestive powers gain strength, boiled onions, roasted potatoes, &c. may be taken. Particular attention should be paid to the cravings of the patient. They are often the calls of nature, and point out the remedy. They are not to be indulged in every thing that their capricious appetites may desire, but when any particular article is eagerly desired, it may be taken in moderate quantity, although it may seem altogether improper.

CONVALESCENCE.

Few are aware of the danger of a relapse in fevers.—The lives of thousands have been lost, apparently for the want of proper care, on recovering from a fever. The stomach and body is extremely weak, and hence will not bear much food nor exercise—in which, convalescent persons are very apt to be indulged.

NURSING.

It will be in vain that the best medicines are given, without a proper nurse, or person, to administer it, and to attend to every duty of her business, and the directions of the physician.

It is the duty of the nurse to pay strict attention to the wants of the patient; to medicine, drink, diet, &c. that they be given in proper quantities and at proper times; that the clothes and bedding of the patient be often changed, and to follow the directions of the physician; for it is always best to follow his directions, or dismiss him at once.

REMARKS.

Enough has already been said to enable any person of common judgment and understanding, to cure all curable cases of fever. As one general cause produces all fevers, so one general course of treatment is proper for all. Yet particular attention should be paid to local symptoms, the habit and temperament of the patient, his peculiarities of constitution, &c. In treating local diseases, care should be taken not to give medicines that act too strongly upon some particular organ that may have been previously weakened or diseased. Notwithstanding these general rules are sufficient in common cases, it may be proper and useful to give a more particular description of the particular divisions, or types, of fever.

Intermittent Fever, or Fever and Ague.

[Febris Intermittens.]

The title of intermittent, is applied to that kind of fever which consists of a succession of paroxisms, between each of which there is a distinct and perfect intermission from febrile symptoms. These paroxisms and remissions vary in their occurrence. They sometimes occur once in twenty-four hours; in other cases, once in forty-eight; and in others, but once in three or four days. Sometimes two or three fits, or paroxisms, occur in one day, and then intermit for one, two, three, or four days; but these variations are only shades of difference in the same disease, and all proceed from the same cause.

CAUSES.

The principal exciting cause of this disease, is the effluvia arising from stagnant water, when acted upon by heat, and from vegetable putrefaction. Drinking impure, or stagnant water, is also among the greatest exciting causes. This disease is also caused by debility, produced by a poor, watery diet, damp houses, evening dews, lying upon damp ground, watchings, fatigue, depressing passions of the mind, &c.

When persons remove from a high to a low country, they are frequently seized with intermittent fevers; and to such the disease is most likely to prove fatal. Hence will be seen the propriety of persons thus removing, being very careful not to be exposed to the night air; as, in such situations, it is much more injurious than in the day time.

SYMPTOMS.

This disease may be divided into the cold, the hot, and sweating stages. The cold stage comes on with pain of the head, limbs, and loins; coldness of the extremities; stretching; yawning; sometimes sickness and vomiting, succeeded by cold, shivering, and violent shaking. After a longer or shorter continuance of shivering, the heat of the body returns gradually, and by transient flushes, which is soon succeeded by a steady, dry, and burning heat. The skin, which was pale and constricted, becomes swollen, red, and very sensible; the pulse hard and quick; thirst great; urine high colored. A moisture at length breaks out on the face, and becomes general; the heat falls to its ordinary standard; the pulse become less frequent, more full, and free; the urine deposites a sediment; the action of the bowels is natural; respiration, or breathing, is easy, and all the functions are restored to their natural order; when, after a specific interval, the paroxism returns, and performs the same successional evolutions.

TREATMENT.

If the attack be light, it may be thrown off by giving freely of the alterative powders, and vegetable elixir, to raise the internal heat; the cathartic pills, No. 69, to cleanse the stomach; and the bitters to restore the digestive powers, and invigorate the system. But if the symptoms are violent, the regular course must be taken, viz: raise the heat in the stomach; then apply the vapor bath; give the injection and emetic, and strengthen the system. There are few diseases in which a patient is more liable to a relapse, and which often happens after a lapse of several weeks, or even months. Hence the importance of continuing the use of medicine until a thorough cure is effected, and the system well strengthened. The patient should be supported by a nutritious diet.

PREVENTION.

To prevent attacks of the ague, or their recurrence when cured, care should be taken to avoid the direct influence of the sun, and particularly the damp air of evening and morning. Flannel, worn next the skin, is very beneficial.

If fires are kept burning in the sitting rooms in the morning and evening during the prevalence of these unhealthy vapors, it will be found useful, by rarifying the air and keeping the walls dry.

It will also be very beneficial to take occasionally such medicines as promote the digestion, regulate the bile, and neutralize the acidity, or sourness. For this purpose, take of the stomach bitters, No 73, the neutralizing mixture, No. 88, and alterative powders, No. 1; and an emetic occasionally will be found highly beneficial.

If the above directions were observed by emigrants settling on low lands, and near marshes, the danger of their being attacked by intermittent and other fevers, would be lessened in a great degree.

Remittent Fever—(Febris Remittens.)

By a remittent fever, is to be understood that modification of fever which abates, but does not go entirely off before a fresh attack ensues; or in other words, where one paroxism succeeds another so quickly, that the patient is never without some degree of fever.

The causes and symptoms of a remittent fever, are very similar to those of an intermittent, attended with severe pain in the back and legs. The fever continues a short time, then a gentle perspiration breaks out, and the fever abates, or goes off imperfectly. This remission continues, perhaps, not more than an hour or two. The fever then commences again as severe as before, and perhaps worse. In warm climates, the remissions frequently come on as early as the second day; but in cold ones, it frequently does not take place until from the fourth to the sixth or eighth day.

The symptoms of intermittent fever vary, according to the situation and constitution of the patient—likewise the season of the year, and other circumstances. In warm climates, the remittent fever often becomes very violent and dangerous. It assumes a putrid character, and prevails as an epidemic. Such fever attacks the patient suddenly, and with great violence. The remissions occur daily, and the eyes become red, yellow, and watery. It frequently proves fatal in a few days.

BILLIOUS REMITTENT FEVER.

This is another form of remittent fever, attended with vomiting of yellow or billious matter; yellowness of the eyes and skin; the tongue coated with yellow fur, &c.

TREATMENT.

These fevers require much the same treatment as intermittents, viz: cleanse the first passages, remove obstructions, and invigorate the system.

Particular attention should be paid to supporting the patient's strength. For this purpose, give the cream cordial, No. 89, and freely of valerian, to relieve nervous irritation.

There are numerous other divisions and types, as the putrid, typhus, yellow, inflammatory, spotted, scarlet, plague, &c. But the same type of fever assumes so many shades of difference, that further descriptions might only tend to involve the prescriber in a labyrinth of perplexity. The following hint, however, may not be amiss: In violent attacks, the most active measures should be taken; and in putrid fevers, to prevent the putrescency, or putrefaction of the blood; and in low fevers, to support the strength by the use of cream cordial, good wine, wine whey, &c.

The celebrated Dr. Donaldson, a man of great erudition in the medical science, and a strict adherent to the principles of the old school, and who had travelled over a great part of the world in search of information on this important science, makes the following remarks:—

"I observed the plan of cure followed by the East Indians, in fevers. I saw the practitioners cure the most vehement cases of intermittent and other fevers, in the space of a single day, with such mathematical precision and certainty, as I had never before beheld in any region of the earth, by purging, vomiting and sweating. I perceived that they also cured without knowing the nature of the disease, or the principles of their practice. Their method of treatment consisted in administering a medicine that effectually purged and vomited their patients, who were obliged at the same time to use the steam bath, and drink abundantly of warm teas, until a profuse sweat was produced; and the fever was mechanically broke or reduced, leaving nothing for feeble nature to perform, as the ancient physicians of Europe were accustomed to do many ages before the days of Batellus and Sydenham.

INFLAMMATORY DISEASES.

All the viscera are subject to inflammation. The various symptoms exhibited in this class of diseases, are owing more to the peculiar structure of the inflamed part, than to the exciting cause. Local inflammations cause more or less general fever, and should be treated on general principles.

Inflammation of the Brain.—*(Phrenitis.)*

Phrenitis, is an inflammation of the membranes of the head, or brain, or both. It usually commences with inflammatory fever, flushed face, intolerance of light and sound, head ache, watchfulness, and delirium.

TREATMENT.

Follow the common course of treatment; give the cathartic pills freely. The stimulating injection should be omitted until the stomach and bowels are cleansed by emetics and cathartics; apply the lobelia fomentation, No. 26, freely and often to the head; keep smart draughts to the feet; give sudorifics freely, and endeavor to keep up a brisk perspiration. The patient must be kept from all noise, and from the light.

Mumps—(*Cynanche Parotidea.*)

Mumps are a swelling of the parotid glands of the neck. They become hard, large, and painful, frequently impeding respiration and swallowing. There is generally some fever attending the disease. It usually, however, requires but little medicine. A teaspoonful each of the alterative powders and vegetable elixir, two or three times a day, and a light cathartic, is sufficient; but in case of a recession by taking cold, or otherwise, by which the complaint is thrown on the testicles, or other parts, a free perspiration should be produced, and the parts poulticed with the elm poultice, and treated as other local inflammations.

Quinzy, or Inflammatory Sore Throat.

[Cynanche Tonsillaris.]

This disease is an inflammation of the tonsils, commonly called the almonds of the ear, or the mucus membrane lining the throat. It produces difficulty of swallowing and breathing, accompanied by redness of the tonsils, dryness of the throat, foulness of the tongue, and lancinating pain in the affected parts. The fever increases, the tongue swells, and respiration becomes difficult. It sometimes terminates in suppuration; sometimes by resolution.

TREATMENT.

In the first stages of the disease, give an emetic of the tincture of lobelia, No. 33, or the infusion of the herb. If the swelling is large and painful, steam it with the following preparation:—Take hops, worm-wood, and catnip; boil them in vinegar; cover the vessel with a funnel, and let the patient inhale the steam; add a hot stone occasionally, to keep the steam moderately warm; continue fifteen minutes, and repeat it once in two or three hours, until relief is obtained; bind the herbs on the throat each time the steam is applied; the compound linament, No. 39, may be applied in the early stage of the disease; the throat should be gargled or washed with a tea of bayberry, lily, golden seal, or sumach berries; a mild cathartic may be given occasionally, and a moderate perspiration kept up.

Croup—(*Cynanchcalis Trachealis.*).

This is an acute inflammation of the mucus membrane of the trachea, or wind-pipe, characterized by fever, cough, hoarseness, difficulty of breathing, &c.

TREATMENT.

Give the tincture of lobelia, half a teaspoonful, in May-weed, pennyroyal, or catnip tea, once in fifteen minutes, until it vomits; then give a mild cathartic of oil, elder-flowers, or senna; apply draughts to the feet; then give the following:—Take of the alterative powder one teaspoonful, cough powder half a teaspoonful; add a tea-cup full of boiling water; strain, and sweeten with honey; give a teaspoonful once an hour, if it does not excite too much nausea. The emetic should be repeated according to the urgency of the symptoms, and clysters given occasionally.

Whooping Cough—(*Pertussis.*)

SYMPTOMS.

The whooping cough usually comes on with difficulty of breathing, quick pulse, and other slight febrile symptoms, which are succeeded by hoarseness, cough, and difficulty of expectoration. The cough becomes convulsive, and is attended by a peculiar sound, called a whoop, and is frequently attended with vomiting.

TREATMENT.

If the symptoms are light, give the alterative powders two or three times a day; and the cough powder, mixed with honey or molasses, at night. But if the symptoms are severe, give gentle emetics—the tincture of lobelia in a little warm tea—or take of lobelia herb one teaspoonful, valerian half a teaspoonful; add half a teacupful of warm water; let it infuse; strain, and give from one to two teaspoonfuls once in fifteen minutes till it operates. Emetics cleanse the stomach and relieve the lungs. The expectorant cordial may be given, or the following:—take of skunk cabbage two ounces, lobelia one fourth of an ounce, hoarhound one ounce, boneset half an ounce, molasses one quart; simmer the whole half an hour; stran it, and give one or two teaspoonfuls three or four times a day. Mild cathartics, as cold expressed castor oil, should be given.

Asthma.—*(Asthma.)*

Symptoms.—Attacks of the asthma commonly commence at night. The patient is oppressed with a tightness across the breast, which strongly impedes respiration. For a considerable time his breathing is very difficult, attended with a wheezing noise; speaking is difficult, and there is a propensity to coughing. Finally, the paroxism goes off gradually, and the patient is relieved. When a person has once been attacked, the paroxisms are apt to return, and the patient is frequently troubled with difficulty of breathing during the intervals.

TREATMENT.

During a paroxism, or fit of the asthma, the patient must be placed in an erect position, his feet immersed in warm water, or the vapour bath applied, and stimulants and sudorifics given, to divert the blood from the lungs and the bronchial vessels; give of the tincture of lobelia from one to three teasponfuls, and repeat it until relief is obtained.

This medicine (lobelia) produces the most astonishing effects in this complaint. It is no sooner taken into the stomach, than the tension and spasm are removed, by dislodging collections of mucus in the bronchial vessels, and thereby giving free admission of air into the lungs; and it is invariably attended with a salutary effect.

Having suspended the paroxism, the next step is to effect a radical cure. For this purpose let the patient continue the use of the tincture of lobelia, in doses of from half to a teaspoonful every night; give freely of the alterative powders, and the pulmonary syrup or expectorant cordial.

Inflammation of the Lungs.—*(Pneumonia.)*

SYMPTOMS.

Inflammation of the lungs comes on with pain in the chest or side, great difficulty of breathing when lying down, with a dryness of the skin, cough, thirst, &c. If relief is not afforded in time, and the inflammation proceeds with such violence as to threaten suffocation, the vessels of the neck become swelled, the face purple, and effusions of blood take place in the lungs, which deprive the patient of life; it also terminates by suppuration and gangrene.

TREATMENT.

The most prompt means, should be used to reduce the inflammation and remove the disease by resolution, or by preventing suppuration. In this, as well as in other diseases, it will be necessary in the first stage to produce a free perspiration, by making use of the vapor bath, and administering sudorific medicines; the patient should be kept in a profuse sweat for several hours; it may then be moderated, but should be continued gently for twenty-four hours, or longer; give the infusion of lobelia in small doses, sufficient to produce sickness at the stomach. When the arterial excitement is abated, give an emetic. It will be found serviceable to inhale the steam of bitter herbs. The tension of the lungs is thus removed, and the mucus expectorated with more ease. It may be repeated two or three times a day, or oftener. The cough powder may be given to assist expectoration.—Slippery elm, or flax-seed tea, may be drank freely. If the cough remains troublesome after the inflammation has subsided, give the pulmonary syrup or pulmonary cordial.

Pleurisy.—(*Pleuritis.*)

Pleurisy is an inflammation of the pleura, or membrane that lines the thorax.

SYMPTOMS.

This disease appears with the general precursors of fever, attended with a violent pricking pain in one side, and coughing. The pain is sometimes so severe as to impede respiration. The matter which is raised is streaked with blood. The pulse is remarkably strong and hard.

TREATMENT.

In this, as in all cases of acute inflammation, the most active measures should be taken to produce and establish copious perspiration. Give the sudorific powders in an infusion of catnip. Apply the bitter fomentation, or compound yest poultice to the side.

Inflammation of the Diaphragm.—(*Paraphrentis.*)

This disease is an inflammation of the diaphragm, or midriff, which divides the thorax from the abdomen.

SYMPTOMS.

There is very violent pain at the lower part of the breast-bone, and under the short ribs, striking through to the back; breathing difficult and frequent; sickness, hiccough; pulse quick and hard. It resembles pleurisy in its leading symptoms.

TREATMENT.

The treatment in this disease the same as in pleurisy.

Inflammation of the Liver.—*(Hepatitis.)*

SYMPTOMS.

The acute species of hepatitis, comes on with a pain in the right side, extending up to the shoulder, which is much increased by pressing upon the part, and is accompanied with a cough, oppression of breathing, nausea, and vomiting of billious matter. The urine is of a deep saffron color. There is a loss of appetite, and costiveness, with a strong, hard pulse; and when the disease has continued for some days, the skin and eyes become tinged with a deep yellow.

TREATMENT.

As in all inflammatory diseases, the first object will be to lessen the determination of blood to the inflamed part, by equalizing the circulation. To effect this, pursue the general course: Apply a fomentation, or poultice, to the side, &c.

Chronic Inflammation of the Liver.

When the disease assumes a chronic character, the symptoms are a dull pain in the right side and shoulder; the stomach disordered; the appetite irregular; a yellow tinge of the skin and eyes, and often swelling in the region of the liver.

TREATMENT.

Give freely of the alterative powders, and alterative syrup; give at bed time, every night, from one to three of the emetic pills; apply a strengthening plaster (No. 63) to the side; give a regular course once or twice a week.

Inflammation of the Spleen.—*(Splenitis.)*

SYMPTOMS.

It is characterized by fever, tension, heat, tumor, and pain in the left hypochondrium, or side, increased by pressure. This disease comes on with excessive shivering, succeeded by intense heat and great thirst, the paroxism resembling the fever and ague. If the patient is exposed to the air, the extremities immediately grow cold. If hemorrhage happens, the blood flows from the left nostril. The other symptoms are the same as inflammation of the liver. Like the liver, the spleen is also subject to chronic inflammation, which often happens after agues, &c.

TREATMENT.

The same course of treatment as laid down for inflammation of the liver.

Inflammation of the Intestines.—*Enteritis.*

This dangerous and painful disease is characterized by acute pain in the bowels, which is increased by pressure, and shoots round the navel in a twisting manner. There is obstinate costiveness, tension of the belly, and a vomiting, generally of a billious, dark, or fetid matter, with general febrile symptoms.

TREATMENT.

The febrile symptoms should be treated on general principles—the stimulating injection given, with the addition of slippery elm, and fomentations applied over the abdomen. The drink should be demulcent and diluting, such as slippery elm, flax seed, &c.

Inflammation of the Peritoneum.

An inflammation of the peritoneum, (or membrane that lines the whole internal surface of the abdomen,) is attended with symptoms very similar to those attending inflammation of the bowels; but the bowels are not always costive in this disease. The abdomen is very hard, and extremely tender. This disease may be mistaken for an inflammation of the bowels. It requires much the same treatment. The vapor bath and fomentations are of great importance.

Inflammation of the Kidneys.—*(Nephritis.)*

This disease is characterized by pain in the region of the kidneys, shooting along the course of the ureters, or ducts, that convey the urine from the kidneys to the bladder, with fever, and frequent discharges of urine in small quantity, and high colored ; the thigh feels numb, attended with pain in the groin. This disease frequently assumes the chronic form ; the symptoms are the same as in the acute, but less severe.

TREATMENT.

The first object is to relax the system by producing perspiration. If the pain is violent, give the diuretic decoction, No. 25, and diuretic drops, No. 18 ; apply fomentations over the kidneys, or poultice ; if the disease is of the chronic character, give the diuretic syrup, No. 7, and a strengthening plaster to the back.

Rheumatism.—*(Rheumatismus.)*

Rheumatism is a very painful disease, which affects the muscles and joints, and frequently some of the internal muscles and organs. It is sometimes attended with fever and swelling of the parts, when it is called acute, or inflammatory ; when there is no swelling or inflammatory symptoms, it is termed chronic.

Very alarming and fatal symptoms sometimes follow a recession of rheumatism. It passes to the heart, diaphragm, stomach, bowels, pleura, head, and other parts.

Dr. Cox, of England, states that the numerous cases of organic disease of the heart and pericardium, which he met with in Guy's hospital, were referable to, or connected with rheumatism. All of which symptoms unquestionably arise from a retention of morbid humors in the system.

TREATMENT.

Inflammatory rheumatism should be treated on the general principles laid down for inflammatory, or febrile diseases. Fomentation should be applied, and the inflamed parts bathed with the compound tincture of lobelia, No. 89, or the compound linament, No. 29. Sudorifics should always be given freely.

When the disease assumes the chronic form, it may be cured by taking freely of the alterative powders and vegetable elixir. Bathe the parts as above; but if it is seated on any internal organ, or proves obstinate, the general course must be resorted to. The vapor bath is of great importance in rheumatism.

Gout.—*(Arthritis.)*

The gout is similar to the rheumatism, proceeds from similar causes, and requires similar treatment. It sometimes attacks by spasm, and generally on the feet, or near the extremities. If the local pain or swelling is very acute, a poultice may be applied. The system is always more or less affected. The disease should therefore be treated on general principles.

Consumption.—*(Phthisis Pulmonalis.)*

Pulmonary consumption is characterized by emaciaciation, debility, cough, hectic fever, and purulent expectoration. The causes that produce this disease, are, any thing that debilitates the constitution, or the application of noxious vapors to the lungs by respiration. Hence persons employed in mines, brick-layers, flax and feather dressers, are very subject to this disease. Sudden and severe colds, the retrocession of eruptive diseases, as small pox and measles, in consequence of the humors settling on the lungs, are causes which often produce the disease; and the means used to cure diseases, particularly this, in its premonitory stages, are not among the least causes that produce it—such as bleeding, mercury, blisters, seatons, tartar emetic, &c.

SYMPTOMS.

The incipient, or early symptoms, vary with the cause of the disease, but the following are the general symptoms: It begins with a short, dry cough, that at length becomes habitual, but by which nothing is raised but a frothy mucus. The breathing is difficult; the strength, flesh, spirits, and appetite fail. In this situation, the patient frequently remains for a considerable time. By degrees, the matter which is expectorated becomes more viscid, and assumes a greenish and purulent appearance, sometimes streaked with blood. The pulse is frequently nearly natural in the first stages of the disease, but as it progresses, the pulse becomes full, hard, and quick.—The face becomes flushed, and hectic fever commences. The mouth and throat are slightly inflamed, and beset with apthea, or canker. The feet swell, or bloat; the extremities grow cold; and in some cases delirium takes place some days before the fatal termination of the disease.

TREATMENT.

In the incipient stage of the disease, it may be cured by giving the alterative powders, cough powders, and pulmonary syrup, or expectorant cordial, and an emetic or two. In the more advanced stages, when the patient has become weak, the pulse quick, the expectoration copious, and of a purulent character, the cure is more uncertain, and requires more particular attention. It will be necessary first to allay the febrile excitement, by giving emetics. The tincture of lobelia is generally most suitable. Give the alterative powder by infusion in water, and sweeten and add milk. Give the cream cordial, from a teaspoonful to a tablespoonful once in three hours. The emetic should be repeated every day, or every other day. Drinks of boneset and vervine should be taken. The cough powder may be given to assist expectoration. When the inflammation has subsided in a measure, and the pulse is lowered to eighty or ninety, the pulmonary cordial may be given, from one to three teaspoonfuls, once in three or four hours. The diet should be light and nutritious. Gentian may be used freely in this disease, in the cough, also alterative powders. If the patient is restless, Bateman's drops, or poppy syrup, may be given sparingly.

ERUPTIVE DISEASES.

Most diseases of this class are characterized by fever, nausea, or vomiting; and at a particular time, numerous small eruptions break out on the surface. Most of this class of diseases are also contagious, and attack a person but once.

All the symptoms exhibited, show conclusively, the pathology of fever, as advocated in this work, to be strictly correct. While the contagious matter is in the circulation, all the phenomena of fever are observed; but as soon as the eruptions, the excitive cause, are thrown to the surface, it subsides; and re-appears when such eruptions or humors are absorbed—thus showing, in the plainest possible manner, the nature and cause of fever.

Small Pox.

Small pox is a disease of a contagious nature, marked by febrile symptoms; succeeded by an eruption; and is divided into ***Distinct*** and *Confluent.*

SYMPTOMS.

In distinct small pox, the disease comes on with inflammatory fever, with its attendant symptoms, which increase until the fourth or fifth day. The eruption generally commences on the third day—first on the face, and then successively on the extremities, until the fifth day, when it is fully completed. The fever then abates, or goes off entirely.

The eruption appears first in small, red spots, very little prominent, but by degrees rising into pimples. On the fifth or sixth day, a small vesicle, or bladder, containing an almost colorless fluid, appears on the top of the pimple. For two days, these vesicles increase in breadth only, but on the eighth they become full. The pustules are surrounded by an inflamed margin. As the disease advances, the matter in the pustules becomes first opaque, or cloudy, then white, and at length yellowish. On the eleventh day, the swelling of the face abates, and the pustules are full. On the top of each, a dark spot appears where the matter oozes out, and forms a scab. After some days, both the crust and pustule fall off, leaving the skin a dark red.

Confluent Species.

In the confluent small pox, all the symptoms above mentioned are more severe. Vomiting generally attends.

The eruption appears earlier, and sometimes in clusters, like the measles. Upon the eruption, the fever suffers some remission, but never goes off entirely; and after the fifth day it increases, and continues through the disease. When the pustules are distinct, their margins are not inflamed, and the matter does not acquire the yellow color.

In this species, there is often considerable putresency of the fluids, as appears from the watery vesicles, under which the skin shows a disposition to gangrene, and forms bloody urine, or other hemorrhages—all of which symptoms frequently attend this disease.

In the confluent kind, the danger is always considerable. When the putrid disposition is great, the disease sometimes proves fatal before the eighth day, but generally not until the eleventh, or even fourteenth or seventeenth day.

TREATMENT.

The object of the physician in this disease, as in every other, ought to be to aid the salutary efforts of nature, in eliminating or expelling the morbific or variolous poison. In the commencement of small pox, it will be found necessary to treat it in a considerable degree upon general principles, having in view, at the same time, particular symptoms, as vomiting, costiveness, pain in the head, &c.

Such is the similarity between eruptive and febrile diseases, that it is sometimes difficult to discriminate between them; and if the diagnostic symptoms are ever so well marked, a very similar course of treatment is called for in both. If vomiting predominates, give the neutralizing mixture, or sal eratus in spearmint tea; then give a mild cathartic. Such medicine should be given as will produce a gentle, but not profuse perspiration. Saffron and catnip, of equal parts, may be given. The alterative powders should be given three or four times a day.—White snake root in infusion may be used—the feet bathed in warm water, &c.

For soreness of the throat, and accumulation of mucus and phlegm, give one or two teaspoonfuls of the tincture of lobelia; to be repeated occasionally. The throat may also be gargled with the stimulating or astringent gargles. If the symptoms are urgent, and the eruptions do not appear, give the emetic powder, No. 3, in conjunction with the above, and give the stimulating injection freely.

When there is a great tendency to putrescency in the fluids, or symptoms of the confluent character, give the vegetable elixir, cream cordial, and wine whey. Common yest is also recommended.

The diet should be light vegetable, and particular attention paid to air and cleanliness. After the eruptions are gone, or fallen off, the patient should take an emetic, and use the vapor bath, to cleanse the last relics of the disease from the system.

INOCULATION.

Since inoculation has been introduced, the small-pox, which proved so destructive to former generations, is no more to be dreaded than the fire on the hearth. When the matter is inserted under the skin, a pimple appears about he third day. On the seventh or eighth day, the symptoms of the disease appear, but are quite mild, and require very little medicine.

Cow-pox, or Vaccine Disease.—(*Vaccina.*)

When this disease is produced by inoculation, it is very mild. The following circumstances are deserving of attention in inoculating for the cow-pox.

That the matter with which we inoculate be not taken later than the ninth day.

That the fluid be perfectly transparent, as it is not to be depended on when it becomes opake and yellow.

That the matter taken should be dried gradually and thoroughly before it is laid aside for use, when it is not employed immediately, or in a fluid state.

That the punctures with the besmeared lancet be made as superficially as possible, and only one in the same arm.

It may be proper to remark, that if there is any herpetic eruption on the skin, the inoculation will not be likely to succeed well.

Chicken, or Swine Pox.

SYMPTOMS.

The eruptions sometimes appear without any previous illness; at others there are some febrile symptoms three or four days before the eruption. On the first day of the eruption they are red, resemble the small-pox, and may be mistaken for that disease in its mildest form. On the second day the red pimples become small vesicles, containing a colourless fluid, but sometimes a yellow liquor. On the third day the pustules arrive at full maturity; on the fifth day of the eruptions, the pustules are almost dried, covered with a crust, and soon fall off.

TREATMENT.

This disease is usually so mild as not to require any medicine; but if the febrile excitement is high, and the eruption assumes the confluent character, or does not appear, which however is very rare, it may be treated similarly to the small-pox.

Measles.—*(Prubeola.)*

The measles are a highly infectious disease, to which the person who has been once attacked is not again liable.

SYMPTOMS.

The eruption is generally preceded by general uneasiness, shivering, and pain in the head, in adults; but in children, heaviness, sore throat, sickness, vomiting, fever, a swelling about the eyes, inflammation, and a defluxion of sharp tears. The light is oppressive.—There is a serous discharge from the nose, with sneezing. The febrile symptoms increase rapidly, to which succeeds dry cough, oppression of the lungs, pain in the loins, sometimes looseness of the bowels, at others profuse sweating; tongue foul, the thirst great, and high fever. The eruption appears about the fourth or fifth day. On the third or fourth day after the eruption appears, the redness diminishes; the spots, or small pimples dry up; the cuticle peels off, and is replaced by a new one. The symptoms do not go off on the eruption, as in small pox, except vomiting. The cough and head-ache continue, with the weakness and defluxion of the eyes, and a considerable degree of fever. On the ninth or eleventh day, no trace of redness is left, and the skin assumes its wonted appearance; yet if there has not been some considerable evacuation by vomiting, or perspiration, the patient will seldom gain strength immediately; but the cough and fever will increase with new violence, and produce great distress and danger.

In more severe cases, spasms, lethargy, delirium, and twitching of the muscles take place. In violent cases of this disease, putrid symptoms sometimes attend.

TREATMENT.

In mild cases of the measles, a strong tea of saffron, snake-root, or of the alterative powders, with a mild cathartic, as a cathartic or billious pill occasionally, will be sufficient, in addition to keeping comfortably warm. In severe cases, it will be necessary to give emetics, and pursue a course of treatment similar to that laid down for small pox. It is of great importance, after the eruption has dried and peeled off, to give an emetic, and use the vapor bath, as this disease leaves the system in a very morbid state. The patient should continue to take the alterative powders for some days after the termination of the disease.

DROPSICAL DISEASES.

In this class of diseases, there is a preternatural or morbid collection of serous fluid in the cellular membrane in the viscera, and the circumscribed cavities of the body, impeding or preventing the functions of life. It is divided, according to its location, into *hydrocephalus*, *hydrothorax*, *ascites hydrocele*, *ascites ovarii*, *hydrometra*, and *anarsarca*.

Dropsy of the Brain.—*(Hydrocephalus.)*

By dropsy of the head, we understand a collection of water, either between the membranes of the brain, or in the ventricles. When the fluid is contained within the ventricles of the brain, it is called internal; and when between the membranes, external. In this latter case, it is usually of the chronic nature; and water has been known to increase to an enormous quantity, swelling the head to a prodigious size.

SYMPTOMS.

The early symptoms are such as generally attend infantile fever; such as often accompany dentition, or teething, or a disordered state of the stomach or bowels, or the effect of worms, followed by head ache, impatient of light or noise; flushed countenance, redness of the eyes, contracted pupil, tossing of the arms to the head, and occasionally screaming or shrieking without any apparent cause; the pulse grows slower and more irregular; the pupils dilate, and cease to contract on the approach of light; there is a squinting of the eyes; the child falls into a state of insensibility and stupor; the screaming fits occur more frequently, and there is almost constant moaning; the child will often vomit on being raised into an erect posture; any sudden exertion brings on convulsions, and the child dies. If, however, he survives these symptoms, the pulse generally rises again, sometimes to 150, or higher, and is very feeble; the child takes nourishment from inability to reject it; he lies insensible; the face is pale, tongue foul, convulsions or paralysis occur; one side, or limb, is perfectly paralytic; severe inflammation of the eyes sometimes happens, and gangrenous spots appear on the neck, lips, and ears.

The symptoms in the chronic form of the disease, are similar to those of the acute, but less violent, and appear in slower succession.

TREATMENT.

The indications of cure in this disease, are to lessen the inflammatory symptoms by equalizing the circulation, and thus preventing effusions of water, and when water has been collected in, to evacuate it through the medium of the absorbent vessels, by stimulating them to a healthy action.

Febrile symptoms must be treated on general principles, and effectual measures taken to divert the blood from the head to the extremities. Let the feet be bathed often in warm water, and draughts applied; the vapor bath used, the tincture of lobelia given for an emetic, and repeated daily. The lobelia fomentation should be applied to the head once in thirty minutes, or oftener, if the pain appear severe, and there is great heat; it should be cool, or cold. A free perspiration must be produced.—Mild cathartics and injections are very important. A tea of the alterative powders, sweetened, and a little milk added, may be given throughout the disease.

Dropsy of the Abdomen, or Belly.—(*Ascites.*)

By this description of dropsy, we understand a collection of water in the abdomen. The water is generally collected in the sac of the peritoneum, or general cavity of the belly; sometimes it is outside the peritoneum.—Sometimes the water is contained in distinct sacs, and connected with some of the viscera. It is then called *encysted* dropsy.

Causes.—A preternatural collection of serous fluid, in any part of the body, is caused by absorption falling short of exhalation in these cavities; and this effect may be produced, either by increased effusion from the exhalent vessels, or from diminished action of the absorbents; or, in other words, the serous fluid, or water, that is carried into these parts by the exhalent vessels in larger quantities than usual, are not taken up by the absorbents and carried off by urine and perspiration, as they should be in a healthy state. This deficiency arises from cold, and debility of those vessels.

This debilitated state of the system depends on various causes. It may be induced by long continued fevers; by excessive evacuations of any kind; by the several kinds of intemperance; by poor watery diet, repeated bleeding, and the use of mineral medicines. It might be thought that the superabundant fluid would readily pass off by the kidneys as they do in a healthy state; but when the stimulus of well oxiginated blood is wanting, the kidneys become torpid, their action ceases, and the quantity of urine becomes diminished. Dropsies are also produced by local inflammations, as of the pleura, peritoneum, liver, brain, &c.

SYMPTOMS.

This variety of dropsy is often preceded by loss of appetite, sluggishness, dry skin, oppression and fullness of the abdomen, scanty discharge of urine, and costiveness. The abdomen enlarges, and a fluctuation of water may be felt by placing both hands on the abdomen, and pressing alternately with each hand ; the distention and weight will be felt on the side on which the patient lies. If the swelling is equal over the belly, we may presume the water to be in the cavity of the abdomen ; but if it is more in one part, and a tumor is felt, it may be encysted. It is very important to distinguish be tween this species of dropsy, and pregnancy, in females, as the greatest mischief might follow a mistake of this kind. A bloating of the face and feet attends this species of dropsy, but it is not always the case. Gravel, or stone in the bladder, sometimes attends this disease.

TREATMENT.

If the disease is mild, it may be cured by the use of the alterative powders to raise the heat ; the diuretic decoction, or hydragogue drops, to evacuate the water ; an emetic to cleanse the stomach ; and the stomach bitters, to restore the digestive powers. But if the symptoms are severe, it will be necessary to resort to a thorough course of treatment. The patient should be carried through a course of emetics, steaming, and injection, which should be repeated once in from one to three days, and the above medicines given at the same time. This will arouse the dormant energies of the system, and carry off the disease. If the kidneys, or other urinary organs are badly affected, or concretions, as stone or gravel in the bladder, they should be treated as laid down under the head of those diseases.

Dropsy of the Chest.—*(Hydrothorax.)*

By this disease, we understand a collection of water in the pericardium, or in the cavities of the thorax.—Sometimes it is diffused in the cellular texture of the lungs without being deposited in the cavity of the thorax. Occasionally the water is enveloped in small cysts, of a membraneous nature, known by the name of hydatids, which apparently float in the cavity of the thorax; but generally they are connected with, and attached to, the pleura.

Causes.—The causes which give rise to this disease, are pretty much the same as those which produce other kinds of dropsy. In some cases, it exists without any other kind of dropsical affection being present; but it often exists as a part of universal dropsy.

SYMPTOMS.

Hydrothorax, or dropsy of the chest, often comes on with uneasiness at the lower end of the sternum, or breast bone, accompanied with a difficulty of breathing, which is increased by any exertion, and which is always more considerable during the night, or when lying down.—With these symptoms, there is a cough, that is at first dry, but which, after a time, is attended with an expectoration. There is generally more or less pain in the arms, near the shoulders; and in some cases, the patient complains of a pressure in the head, and giddiness on stooping forward.

As the disease advances, which is frequently very slow, the difficulty of breathing increases, and the patient is obliged to sit up, and often keep his mouth open.—The pressure of the water, by its irritating effect upon the membranes, often produces violent paroxisms of pain in the diaphragm, peritoneum, and pleura. Sometimes a sensation of water, floating in the thorax, is felt when changing position. The countenance shows symptoms of great anxiety and suffering. The feet and legs generally swell; an irregular palpitation of the heart, and inequality of the pulse, generally attend this disease.

The progress of hydrothorax to a fatal termination, is regular and certain, when not arrested by proper medical treatment, and is generally reckoned among the incurable diseases. But under proper treatment, it may generally be cured as easily as most other chronic diseases.

TREATMENT.

If the disease appears in its milder form, it may be cured by pursuing the treatment laid down for the early stages, or mild symptoms, of ascites; but if the disease does not yield to this treatment, a more thorough course must be adopted. If the disease is in an advanced stage, the patient weak, and the difficulty of breathing great in consequence of the quantity of water, the following course is generally attended with success:

Give of the alterative powder, a teaspoonful, once in three hours, or an infusion of the powders; give of the hydragogue drops, No. 19, from one to three teaspoonfuls, once in three hours; apply the vapor bath occasionally, and give sudorific infusions freely; endeavor to keep up a brisk perspiration; give the diuretic decoction, No. 25; if the urine is not discharged copiously, or the urinary organs appear dormant, the stimulating injection must be given, and repeated once in two or three hours. If the lungs appear oppressed with phlegm, or mucus, a very gentle emetic, as the tincture of lobelia, may be given in an infusion of boneset; or which is perhaps more safe, the cough powder, may be given. As by degrees the water is evacuated, the patient will be faint and exhausted, or may be suddenly attacked with faintness. Should this be the case, the strength should be supported by the use of the cream cordial, vegetable elixir, wine bitters, &c. Should spasmodic affections of the membranes supervene, the vapor bath, sudorifics, and stimulants, with the nerve powder, should be given.

When the disease is removed, the system should be strengthened by the use of tonics, to prevent a relapse of this, or an attack of some other disease; for it is but to be known that the patient has the dropsy, to know that the blood is in a bad state, and that the system generally is cold and debilitated.

Cellular Dropsy.—*(Anasarca.)*

By anasarea, is to be understood a collection of water in the cellular membrane, which is diffused throughout the body, and which is moistened by the fluid thrown out by the exhalent arteries. The quantity of this fluid may be greatly increased, and form the disease called anasarca. The causes may be the same that produce the other species.

SYMPTOMS.

Anasarea, or cellular dropsy, usually commences in the lower extremities, and first shows itself with a swelling of the feet and ankles, which by degrees ascends, and successively occupies the thighs and trunk of the body. The swelling is soft, and an impression made by the finger remains sometime. When the disease is far advanced, the lungs are oppressed by a collection of water in the cellular membrane. The pulse is generally feeble, and great debility attends.

TREATMENT.

The treatment laid down for dropsy of the thorax and abdomen, is particularly applicable to this species also. It is very important to attend particularly to the excretions by perspiration and urine, and to strengthen and invigorate the system.

The other species of dropsy are *hydrocle*, or *dropsy of the scrotum; ascites ovarii, dropsy of the ovariis; hydrometra*, or *dropsy of the uterus.*

These species all arise from the diminished absorption and excretion, and all require the same general course of treatment.

Epilepsy, or Falling Sickness.—*(Epilepsia.)*

SYMPTOMS.

The premonitory symptoms of this disease, are, languor, head-ache, giddiness, dimness of sight, or flashes of light passing before the eyes, ringing in the ears, coldness of the extremities, &c. but the fit often attacks without any warning. He falls down suddenly, gnashes his teeth, and froths at the mouth ; the convulsive agitations of the body are violent, the eyes are reverted, or rolled back in the head, and the patient frequently presents a horrible spectacle of suffering.

We are told by Dr. Pary, that whatever may be the

primary, or first cause of epilepsy, its immediate cause is an excessive impetus, or pressing of blood in the vessels of the brain.

TREATMENT.

The first object is to remove all sources of irritation, moderate the afflux of blood to the brain, and alter the morbid condition of the nervous system, on which convulsions depend, and strengthen the body. The fits may be relieved by giving the compound tincture of lobelia, in doses of from one to three tablespoonfuls.—This will generally break the fit; then give antispasmodic and nervine medicines, as valerian, skull-cap, antispasmodic syrup, &c. between the occurrence of the fits; give emetics to cleanse the stomach, tonics to strengthen the system, and endeavor to promote perspiration, remove obstructions, and equalize the circulation.

Apoplexy.—*(Apoplexia.)*

Apoplexy is a sudden privation, in some degree, of all the senses and motions of the body, except those of the heart and lungs, attended by stupefaction and snoring. This disease is caused by a pressure of blood, or an extravasation of blood, in consequence of the rupture of a blood vessel, or cold and water in the cavities of the brain. Apoplexy makes its attacks at an advanced period of life; and most usually on those of a corpulent habit, with a short neck, large head, and who lead an inactive life, and use a full diet and strong liquors.

Apoplexy sometimes attacks in the course of other diseases, as fevers, small pox, rheumatism, gout, and whooping cough; and it is a still more frequent consequence of organic diseases of the heart, which retard the blood in its return to the extremities.

SYMPTOMS.

The most usual form of an attack of apoplexy, is after the occurrence of some of the above premonitory symptoms. The patient falls suddenly, deprived of sense and motion, and lies as though in sound sleep. In other cases, the patient is attacked with violent pain in the head, with paleness of the face, sickness, and vomiting;

and in some instances falls in a state resembling syncope, or fainting, and then partially recovers, but finally sinks into a state of perfect lethargy; in other cases, a palsy of one side commences, with loss of speech, and gradually passes into apoplexy.

TREATMENT.

The object in this disease, is, during the paroxism, to suspend or remove it, by recalling the blood from the head to the extremities and surface, and prevent a determination of blood to that organ.

When a person is affected with the symptoms, or attacked with a paroxism, the most prompt and energetic measures must be taken. The patient must be placed in a recumbent position favorable to respiration; all tight bandages, or ligatures, removed; the feet and legs immersed in warm ley-water, or placed over a brisk steam; give copious injections, and if the patient can swallow, an emetic; mild cathartics, in moderate doses; and the alterative treatment should be continued for some time.

Catalepsy.—*(Catalepsia.)*

Catalepsy consists in a temporary suspension of voluntary motion and consciousness. The body always remains in the exact position in which it was when the attack came on. The fit does not generally last but a a short time, and leaves the person as well as before the attack, but it sometimes continues for hours, or even days. Consciousness is not always suspended, and the patient recollects what passes.

TREATMENT.

During the paroxism, friction should be applied over the whole body, and such means used as will promote circulation, perspiration, and digestion; and antispasmodics and restoratives administered with suitable diet and exercise.

Hysterics.—*(Hysteria.)*

Hysterics is characterized by a grumbling noise in the bowels; a sense of suffocation as though a ball was ascending to the throat; stupor, insensibility, convulsions, laughing and crying without any visible cause; sleep interrupted by sighing and groaning, attended with flatulence and nervous symptoms. It is caused by affections of the womb, &c.

TREATMENT.

When the fits are light, a few doses of the alterative powders and valerian, will generally relieve; if the fits are severe, give a tablespoonful of the tincture of lobelia. Apply the bitter fomentation over the abdomen; give injections. If this does not effect a cure, attend to a general alterative course of emetics, steaming, &c. The disease which produces the fits is inflammatory, and should be treated accordingly. It is of special importance to give freely of antispasmodics, as valerian, skullcap, the antispasmodic syrup, &c.

Palsy.—(*Paralysis.*)

Palsy is a disease which principally affects the nervous system, and is supposed to arise from any cause that prevents the flow of the nervous power from the brain; hence tumors, over-distention, effusions, translation of morbid matter by a suppression of usual evacuations, pressure made on the nerves by uxation, wounds, fractures, or other injuries, may be reckoned among the causes.

It is attended with an entire or partial loss of sensation and motion of the part affected. There are innumerable degrees of paralytic affection, from the weakness and torpor of a finger, up to the complete apoplexy, in which sense and motion perish throughout the whole body.—To enumerate each of these, would be useless.

TREATMENT.

In case the patient is suddenly and violently attacked, the same course must be pursued as in apoplexy—steaming applied generally, or locally, and stimulating applications, such as the vegetable elixir, compound tincture of lobelia, with friction; and such other means as promote and equalize the circulation, comprise the treatment for this disease.

St. Vitus' Dance.—(*Chocara Sancti Viti.*)

This is a singular disease, characterized by a twitching action of the muscles of one side, or the whole system—it may be primary, or symptomatic. It may arise from the natural debility and extreme irritibility of the patient. This state of the system may be induced by a morbid state of the stomach, teething, worms, acidity in the bowels, violent affections of the mind, &c.

SYMPTOMS.

The contortions and gesticulations of the patient, render him a singular object of observation. All the muscles of voluntury motion are more or less affected—those of the face, neck, and limbs, particularly suffer. The hands and arms are in constant motion; he can grasp no object steadily, and makes on the whole a ludicrous and yet painful appearance.

TREATMENT.

Enquire after the exciting causes, and remove them, and strengthen the system; and as the stomach and bowels are generally in a morbid condition, emetics, injections, and laxitives, are the first medicines—then tonics, antispasmodics, and nervines.

Cholera Morbus.—(*Cholera Morbus.*)

Cholera Morbus is a disease of the stomach and bowels, characterized by vomiting and purging, with severe griping and cramps in the stomach, abdomen, and extremities. It is caused by an excess of morbid bile, or acid, in the stomach, connected with cold.

TREATMENT.

As the exciting causes of this disease are an excess of acid, or vitiated bile, the first indications, therefore, is to destroy this offending matter. For this purpose, give the neutralizing mixture, No. 88, in spearmint tea, or give saleratus in small quantities; administer the stimulating injection, with the addition of saleratus, a piece the size of a common large bean, and repeat them once in fifteen minutes, or according to the symptoms; chicken broth is also useful to allay the irritibility of the stomach. If these means do not relieve, give an emetic; give freely of the vegetable elixir; if the surface appears cold, or the skin contracted, bathe with cayenne pepper and spirits, or elixir. After urgent symptoms are relieved, give the antidysenteric cordial, and neutralizing mixture, and alterative powders.

Water Brash.—*(Pyrosis.)*

The attacks of pyrosis generally come on in the morning; the first symptom is pain in the stomach, with a sense of constriction, and is followed by eructation of considerable quantity of a thin, watery fluid, sometimes sour, at others insipid, or tasteless; sometimes it appears like jelley; after considerable eructation, the fit goes off; it however returns often, and is very troublesome.

TREATMENT.

The neutralizing mixture and alterative powders, are sufficient to effect a cure. It is sometimes necessary to give an emetic, and the stomach bitters in addition.

Indigestion.—*(Dyspepsia.)*

Dyspepsia is a derangement of the digestive functions, occasioning an interruption of the organs, or viscera, concerned in the process of digestion.

"Gregory, a very eminent writer of the old school, says:—Long as it has been made the subject of inquiry by medical authors, it remains involved in much obscurity. The pathology of the disease is little understood; the method of its treatment is still imperfectly known; and the most remarkable diversity of opinions are entertained with regard to the extent to which it influences the production of other diseases."

Causes.—The proximate causes of dyspepsia, may depend on a morbid state of the glands subservient to digestion. The saliva may be deficient—the gastric juice may be deficient, or secreted in too large quantity, or vitiated, whereby the coats of the stomach become enveloped, in a thick, tenacious mucus; the bile may be vitiated, and interfere with the digestive process. Dyspepsia may arise from a morbid condition of the nerves of the stomach, or from general torpor, or defect of the whole nervous system.

The remote or intermediate causes of dyspepsia, are from occasionally overloading, habitual over-feeding, and indulging in spirituous liquors, or wine; want of exercise; from excessive or long continued evacuations; from cold, and from anxiety of mind.

Dyspepsia may be produced by the sympathetic affection of the stomach with other parts, as of habitual costiveness, of chronic disease of the liver, or spleen, functional disturbance of the uterus, obscure disease of the kidneys, chronic affection of the bronchia, &c. Dr. E. Smith says, the real cause of the dyspepsia, is a foul, cold state of the stomach, and that there is no cure without cleansing and warming it, and restoring the tone of the system generally. This, briefly, comprehends the whole.

SYMPTOMS.

When the disease originates in the stomach, the symptoms are nausea, pain in the epigastrium, heart-burn, a sense of fulness, distention, or weight in the stomach, acid, or fetid eructations, occasionally vomiting, a sinking sensation, or fluttering in the stomach, and loss of appetite. Other symptoms are costiveness, an irregular state of the stomach and bowels, debility, lassitude, &c.

TREATMENT.

The objects to be kept in view in the treatment of dyspepsia, are: 1st, to obviate the several exciting causes of it; 2d, to expel from the stomach the several offending agents; 3d, to obviate costiveness; 4th, to improve the tone of the stomach, and remove urgent or distressing symptoms. With a view of fulfilling the first indications, the patient must abstain from every exciting cause which appears to have given rise to the disease, whether in eating or drinking, or any other irregularity; and if this disease appears to have been induced by a disease of some other part, as the liver, spleen, kidneys, or other viscera, these local diseases should be treated as laid down under their respective heads.

For removing from the stomach the offending agents,

emetics must be administered ; they prove very beneficial in dyspepsia ; first, by evacuating the offending matter ; and second, by imparting new tone and vigor to the stomach and whole system.

The stomach and wine bitters may be given ; the neutralizing mixture is a very important medicine, to neutralize the acidity or sourness of the stomach. To restore the tone of the bowels, injections are important. The alterative powders, and vegetable elixir, should be given freely.

When the symptoms are not severe, nor of long standing, the disease may be cured by giving the alterative powders and elixir, an emetic or two, the stomach, or wine bitters, and neutralizing mixture.

Convulsions, or Fits.—*(Spasmi.)*

The term convulsion is usually applied to all kinds of spasmodic affections, such as hysterics, epilepsy, &c. But it is the design here to speak of those fits, or convulsions, which occur in children, and sometimes in adults, which assume no specific character, and when they proceed from the eruption being retained or thrown back in eruptive diseases, from acrid matter in the stomach, as various kinds of poison ; or from flatulence, teething, worms, sudden emotions of the mind, as fear, anger, &c.

SYMPTOMS.

Previous to the attack, there is often debility, languor, and unnatural appearance of the countenance and eyes ; at other times, there is a sudden accession, or attack.—The patient is seized with a sudden spasmodic affection, shakes violently, and falls down and remains senseless, with involuntary motions ; twitching of the muscles ; the jaws set tight ; the eyes fixed, and a discharge of saliva from the mouth.

TREATMENT.

Where the attack is violent, give the tincture of lobelia ; to a child, a teaspoonful, or upwards ; to an adult, from one to three tablespoonfuls ; or the compound tincture of lobelia, which is more powerful. If the jaws are closed, introduce the medicine between the cheek and teeth, by means of a phial, or otherwise; and when it strikes the roots of the tongue, the mouth will open; then give warm, sudorific drink. If this does not relieve, give the stimulating injection, and put the patient into the vapor bath. When the spasms are relieved, enquire into the exciting causes, and treat them accordingly.—Cramp in the stomach, and other parts, should be treated on the same principles.

Heart Burn.—*(Cardiolgia.)*

This disease is an uneasy sensation in the stomach, attended with a kind of burning and distention of the stomach, nausea, retching, and other unpleasant symptoms. It is caused by acrid humors contained in the stomach, or the fumes arising from them.

TREATMENT.

The neutralizing mixture and alterative powders are generally sufficient, but an emetic is sometimes necessary.

Canker, Thrush, or Sore Mouth.—*(Apthea.)*

Canker is among the worst diseases that afflict mankind, especially the young. It generally affects the throat and mouth first, and frequently extends through the stomach and bowels; and is the immediate or remote cause of many other diseases. It is supposed to be caused by retention of cold, acrid humors, turned upon the mouth, stomach, and intestines.

SYMPTOMS.

The apthea is generally preceded by an uneasy sensation, or burning in the stomach, which increases gradually; after sometime, small pimples show themselves on the tongue and throat, which increase, and the mouth becomes very sore and raw; the skin is dry, the pulse small, countenance pale, and extremities cold. It is frequently attended with diarrhœa, loss of appetite, &c. Canker, by eating off small blood vessels, causes spitting blood, and discharges of blood by stool.

TREATMENT.

The first object in the treatment of canker, is to cleanse the stomach by giving emetics; then give a tea of bayberry bark and red raspberry leaves, sweetened with honey; give the alterative powders, or the infusion with milk, sweetened; or if the above cannot be obtained, give a tea of witch hazel, white lily, hemlock bark, sumach bark, or berries, blue scabish, gold thread, or golden seal. Emetics are very important in this disease, as they throw the offending matter off, without passing through the bowels. Injections should be given to clear the bowels.

Vomiting.—*(Emesis.)*

When vomiting occurs spontaneously from irritibility of the stomach, without appearing to depend on any other disease, or when it continues too long after giving an emetic, it may generally be relieved by one or two doses of the neutralizing mixture, and a little spearmint tea, soda, peppermint, burnt corn, and sage, in infusion, may be given. The tincture of common pig weed is also an excellent preparation to stop vomiting. If these means fail, a gentle emetic should be given—the tincture or infusion of lobelia. Bateman's drops are often highly beneficial; as is also a mustard plaster, applied over the stomach.

Dysentery.—*(Dysenteria.)*

This is an affection or inflammation of the alimentary canal, characterized usually by nausea, pain, fever, tensemus, with fetid mucus, or bloody evacuations, and is sometimes contagious.

Causes.—Dysentery may be caused by whatever obstructs the perspiration. Morbid humors are thrown with the blood upon the intestines, causing all the phenomena of the disease. It sometimes appears to be caused by contagion, becoming epidemic in jails, camps, hospitals, ships, &c. It may depend on a putrid acrimony generated in the system. The immediate cause of dysentery appears to be the existence of a corroding acid lodged in the intestines, which produces canker and inflammation, and the attendant symptoms of dysentery. This acid is supposed to be of the nitrous kind.

TREATMENT.

The object in this disease is to neutralize the acid which produces it, cleanse the bowels, and stop the supernatural discharge. For this purpose, give the neutralizing mixture, No. 94, or cordial, No. 88, sufficient to operate as a mild cathartic, and repeat it; then give the antidysenteric cordial. Injections are of the utmost importance in dysentery; the stimulating, or common injections, may be given; saleratus, or soda, should always be added to the injection. If the stomach appear irritable, or the above means do not effect a cure, an emetic must be given. The vegetable elixir should always be given freely in this disease.

Billious Cholic.—*(Cholica.)*

This species of cholic seems to depend upon a superabundance of vitiated or morbid bile in the stomach and bowels, which produces spasmodic contraction of the abdomenial muscles, and distention of the stomach by wind.

SYMPTOMS.

The billious cholic generally attacks the patient violently. It generally appears with nausea, vomiting of yellowish, or billious matter; a bitter taste in the mouth; circumscribed pain about the navel; sometimes the most excruciating pain all over the abdomen; obstinate costiveness, with frequent desire to stool; the skin is generally very dry.

TREATMENT.

In the less violent attacks, it will be sufficient to give the neutralizing mixture, to allay the irritibility of the stomach; then give the infusion of the alterative powders, with the vegetable elixir, in large and repeated doses, and apply the bitter fomentation over the abdomen; but when the symptoms are severe, it is necessary to excite a perspiration; for it is often the case that the most powerful medicines will have no effect until it is produced, when the pain will cease, and the patient fall asleep. Injections are of the greatest importance in this disease. There is no disease in which their sovereign power to remove disease, and the preference this class of medicines hold over all others for removing complaints of the bowels, is so clearly demonstrated as in billious cholic. They constitute, with the above means for warming the system, and exciting perspiration—the treatment for billious cholics. When the urgent symptoms are reliev-ed, it will be necessary to give an emetic or cathartic, with bitters to correct the secretion of bile.

All the other species of cholic should be treated upon the same principle, as cold, obstruction, and spasm, are the exciting causes.

Vomiting Blood.—*(Hematamacis.)*

By this disease, we understand a discharge of blood from the mouth, attended by retching and vomiting. It may be produced by any cause which excites a strong determination of blood to the stomach, or from debility, or relaxation of certain blood vessels; and, which is perhaps oftener the case, from canker in the stomach.

TREATMENT.

As this disease arises from a relaxation, or opening, by some means, of the blood vessels of the stomach, or neighboring parts, astringents will of course be the first medicine. Of these, the essence of whipsiwog is, perhaps, superior to all others. It may be given in doses of from five to fifteen or twenty-five drops, with vegetable elixir, and repeated according to the symptoms. If the essence is not at hand, the expressed juice, or infusion of the herb, may be used; or other astringents, as bayberry, hemlock, lily, scabish, &c. After the effusion is stopped, it is necessary to inquire into the exciting cause, and treat it accordingly. Coughing and spitting blood must be treated on the same principle.

Bleeding at the Nose.—*(Epistaxis.)*

This is a very common complaint. It is very trouble-some, and sometimes dangerous, producing great debility, and occasioning other diseases, from the habitual loss of blood. When bleeding from the nose is not easily stopped, a pledget of lint, or cloth dipped in the essence of whipsiwog, stuffed in the nostril, or pulverized bayberry bark, or other astringents, will generally stop it. If these means fail, let the feet be immersed in warm water, and apply a cold application to the head, and endeavor to equalize the circulation. Smoked beef, dried and grated fine, is extolled very highly for curing this complaint. The powder of common nettles, beth root, &c. are recommended.

Bleeding from wounds may be stopped by the same means recommended for bleeding at the nose.

Involuntary or excessive discharge of Urine. *(Diabetes.)*

This disease is characterized by large quantities of urine, and often by an involuntary discharge of the same. It is accompanied with great debility, costiveness, fever, voracious appetite, emaciation, and a large proportion of saccharine, and other matter, which is voided in a larger quantity than that of the food and drink. It may be caused by intemperance, or from cold, poor diet, diuretic medicines of an improper kind, and an impoverished state of the blood, which may arise from various causes.

TREATMENT.

The object in this disease will be to restore the tone of the system, which may be effected by restorative medicines. The general restorative and alterative course must be pursued. The red mulberry bark of the root is a very valuable article in this disease. A dry and nutritious diet is one of the greatest auxiliaries in the cure of this disease.

Jaundice.—*(Icterus.)*

This disease is characterized by a yellowness of the skin and eyes, dull pain in the head, drowsiness, lassitude, &c. It is caused by an obstruction of the bile in its passage into the duodenum, and is taken into the circulation.

TREATMENT.

When the disease is light, a few potions of the cathartic pills, with the use of the stomach bitters, will cure ; but if obstinate, give emetics and powders.

Worms.—(*Vermes.*)

The symptoms, which are attributed to the effects of worms, are caused, in a great measure, by a disordered state of the stomach ; which is induced by eating unripe fruit, raw herbs, and indigestible matter.

SYMPTOMS.

The common symptoms of worms, are paleness of the face, flushing of the cheeks, itching of the nose, starting, grinding of the teeth when asleep, swelling of the upper lip, and loss of appetite ; at other times, a very craving appetite, a sour stinking breath, a hard swelled belly, great thirst, the urine frothy, or whitish, griping or cholic pains, dry cough, unequal pulse, palpitation of the heart, fainting, choking, drowsiness, cold sweats, palsy, epileptic fits, with many other singular nervous symptoms ; vomiting also frequently attends.

TREATMENT.

The treatment for worms generally consists in such means as will cleanse and warm the stomach, and restore the digestive functions. This course will generally relieve all the symptoms of the disease. To effect these objects, give first an emetic ; then give an infusion of the alterative powders, with the vegetable elixir, and the following bitters : Take balmony one ounce, poplar bark one ounce ; add half a pint boiling water ; then strain, and add one ounce elixir ; give from one to three or four teaspoonfuls, three times a day ; if vomiting attend, give the following—take new milk, half a pint ; add one tablespoonful hot ashes ; strain, and give one or two tablespoonfuls, and repeat it ; then give the emetic ; or take carolina pink and senna, equal parts ; steep and give occasionally, till it operates as a cathartic, and then give the bitters; but if the symptoms are severe, the emetic and injection must be given immediately.

Head-Ache.—(*Cephalalgia.*)

The head-ache arises from various causes. When it arises from a foul state of the stomach, the treatment belongs exclusively to the stomach. When it is of a nervous character, nervine and antispasmodic medicines may be given; when it depends on an excessive determination of blood to the head, the feet should be bathed or soaked in warm water, and proper means used to equalize the circulation. When there does not appear to be any urgent symptoms connected with the head-ache, bathing the crown every morning with cold water, has a good effect. The cephalic snuff, No. 4, is very useful in most cases of head-ache.

SCALDS, OR BURNS.

In the first instance of a burn, or scald, apply a cloth, wet with cold water; or if there be any cloth on the part, as a stocking, or sleeve, pour on cold water immediately, and wrap it close, to prevent the effect of the air. Whenever the smart increases, apply more water. If the burn is large and severe, give the alterative powders, to prevent its affecting the stomach. When the skin is broken, or there is any considerable inflammation, apply the detergent poultice, No. 47; change it once in twelve hours, and wash the sore with soap-suds, and then with an infusion of strong tea of the detergent powders. When the inflammation has abated, apply the burn-ointment, No. 55, or green salve, No. 53, and wash as above. Should fungus, or proud flesh appear, apply lobelia seed, pulverized, or the vegetable caustic.

FREEZING.

Freezing produces the same effect on the human body, as a burn or scald, and should be treated on the same principles, viz: Apply cloths, wet with cold water, to remove the frost, and then proceed as above.

GRAVEL, OR STONE.

This disease is caused by a morbid state of the kidneys, which may arise from strains, or other causes, and which produce a chronic disease of these organs; in consequence of which, their functions become deranged, and there is secreted, with the urine, a morbid matter which lodges in the bladder, and forms hard concretions, or stones, which sometimes gain the weight of a pound, or upwards. These stones are generally composed of a very fine sand, and hard as emery. This sand is combined with a glutinous substance to form the stone.

SYMPTOMS.

The symptoms of this distressing disease, are, at first, a difficulty in voiding urine—a partial suppression of that evacuation. As the disease advances, these difficulties increase, attended with debility, and excruciating pain in voiding urine, which sometimes extends down along the thighs, and towards the anus, with a sense of weight in the bladder. These are generally attended with some febrile symptoms, loss of appetite, thirst, &c. Dropsy of the abdomen frequently attends this disease.

TREATMENT.

This disease has long been considered as incurable by medicine, and the lithotomic operation, or cutting to remove the stone, has generally been resorted to. This operation is, however, attended with great pain and danger, and with no certainty of a cure, as another concretion of the same character may form, if the patient survive the operation of removing the first. It is therefore certainly desirable to remove the cause and effect at the same time, and thus cure the disease, which can be effected as certainly as in almost any other disease.

The first object in the treatment of this complaint, is, to remove the febrile symptoms, and attend to the secretions and excretions. For this purpose, give the emetic and stimulating injection, and apply the steam freely; then give the diuretic syrup, No. 7, and decoction, No. 25. The following tincture has a surprising effect in dissolving these concretions: Take of blood root one ounce, white violets, root and top, one ounce, gin one pint: give half a wine-glass full three times a day. If the pain and irritation about the bladder is great, apply the bitter fomentation. The stimulating injection is of the greatest importance in this disease, as there is no other means of carrying medicine so near the seat of the disease. The patient should be carried through the same course laid down for febrile diseases, every day, or every other day, taking the above medicines, and take the alterative powders during the intervals. If the above course of treatment is thoroughly attended to, it seldom fails of effecting a radical cure.

CHILBLAINS.

This is a very troublesome disease, which generally affects the hands and feet. It is caused by exposing the feet to extreme cold, and suddenly warming them, and by freezing, and going with the feet long wet and cold. This causes swelling, inflammation, and an intolerable itching and burning.

TREATMENT.

Soaking the feet in weak ley-water, with the addition of a little flour of slippery elm bark; or wheat bran will generally relieve the heat and swelling; then bathe with the elixir and emmolient ointment; and if this does not relieve, apply the elm or yest poultice, and then bathe as above.

CORNS AND CALLUSES.

These troublesome excrescences may be cured by soaking the parts thoroughly, removing the dead skin, applying the emmolient ointment, and repeating the operation.

TOOTH-ACHE.

The tooth-ache may generally be relieved by holding the elixir hot in the mouth, and then applying the tooth-ache drops. Cantharides or, (Spanish flies,) mixed with lard, and put into the tooth, will sometimes stop the pain entirely.

Hydrophobia, or Canine Madness.

Causes.—In the human system, it is always the result of a specific contagion, or poison, derived from the bite of an animal laboring under the disease. The poison appears to be confined to the saliva and blood, and can only be communicated by the saliva to the blood.

SYMPTOMS.

At some uncertain period after the bite, a painful tension, redness, and heat, attack the part bitten, and at the same time darting pains and spasms arise in it. The patient is seized with languor, lassitude, anxiety, twitching of the tendons, nervous irritation, disturbed sleep, &c. These symptoms increase; a great aversion to water and other liquids—the sight of which will excite spasms, and an ejection of frothy saliva frequently attends. During the paroxism, the patient often exhibits a disposition to bite, and presents a frightful appearance. Respiration becomes hurried, and gasping convulsions and death end the scene.

TREATMENT.

It is of the utmost importance in this disease to attend to the first symptoms; and if the patient has suspicion that the animal by which he is bitten is affected with hydrophobia, he may apply the remedies laid down for the cure which will effectually prevent its appearance. For this purpose, give the alterative powders and emetic pills for one or two days; then give a thorough course of emetic and injection, and apply the vapor bath; then give the cathartic pills in large doses, and repeat this course from one to three times; then continue the use of the powders and pills for some time; give also of valerian and skull-cap; bathe the wound with the tincture of lobelia.

If the symptoms begin to appear, give the alterative powders; and then attend to the alterative course, i. e. emetic, &c. Give freely of skull-cap. This is used as a specific in this disease by some practitioners.

Cancer and Schirrus.

A hard tumor, or schirrus, is considered as the occult

or primary stage of cancer. A cancer is the worst kind of ulcer.

SYMPTOMS.

A cancer usually begins with a swelling in the gland, unaccompanied by any pain, or any discoloration of the skin. It gradually increases both in size and hardness. In process of time, it is affected with lancinating pains, as though a sharp pointed instrument was entering the tumor, and with various swellings of the neighboring parts and veins. Sometimes the tumor remains in an indolent or schirrous state for a considerable time; but in other instances, it proceeds on to suppuration, and forms an ulcer with great rapidity. As the disease advances, the parts frequently adhere to the bone, and the skin adheres very closely and firmly to the tumor. Sometimes the tumor assumes a purple or reddish appearance. If the ulceration is extensive, some parts will be in a state of sloughing—others will send forth granulations of spongy flesh, generally of a bright red color.

TREATMENT.

If the cancer is in a state of tumor, apply the following plaster:—Take of poke root, half a bushel; obtain the strength by boiling; boil to the consistence of tar; then add five pounds of fresh butter, three pounds of beeswax, and one pound of mutton tallow; simmer slowly until the water is evaporated, and it is fit for use.

Let this plaster be spread on linen and applied to the tumor, and removed once in twelve or twenty four hours. Every night on going to bed, steam the tumor and neighboring parts, with a decoction of the bitter fomentation. Give at the same time the following syrup: Take yellow dock root two pounds, bitter-sweet bark of the root two pounds; boil till the strength is obtained; boil to one gallon, and add sugar; take a wine-glass full three times a day, and take freely of the emetic pills; an emetic should be given once or twice a week, and the general alterative course pursued. If the plaster does not cause sloughing or ulceration, the vegetable caustic may be applied with each plaster. After ulceration takes place, apply the sorrel plaster, No. 67, or cancer plaster,

No. 65; if the inflammation is high, apply the alkaline, or elm poultice, and the sorrel plaster alternately; the compound ointment is also a good application for healing cancerous ulcers, after the application of caustics and plasters. Ferris' plaster is also excellent for discussing cancerous tumors. When the tumor is small, or but a small ulcer, apply the caustic; and then the sorrel plaster and compound ointment will generally cure.

SCROFULA.

This disorder consists in hard indolent tumors, of the conglobate glands, in various parts of the body, but particularly in the neck, behind the ears, and under the chin, which, after a time, degenerate into ulcers, from which is discharged a white curdled matter, somewhat resembling the coagulum of milk.

SYMPTOMS.

Among the earliest characteristic symptoms, are swelling of the glands. Such tumors sometimes continue for a long time unattended by any pain or constitutional disturbance. Sometimes they subside spontaneously, but generally suppuration of an imperfect kind takes place. The ulcers heal slowly, leaving ragged and unsightly scars, and are succeeded by other tumors which run a similar course. In this course, the disease is often continued for years, until at length the constitution strengthening, throws it off, or it appears in some of its more severe and dangerous forms.

The scrofulous abscess is distinguished by its jagged and uneven sides. The pus, or matter, instead of having a bland, uniform cream-like appearance, is thin or ichorous, and mixed with curdy flakes. The tumors and ulcers assume various appearances.

This disease generally attacks children of light skin and hair, blue eyes, ruddy cheeks, and very fine soft skin. These are by some authors, marked as constitutional symptoms of the disease.

TREATMENT.

When the disease attacks with pain, swelling, and

inflammation, the following poultice must be applied:— Take dragon turnip—[wild turnip]—if green, or fresh, bruise—add a little water, and sufficient slippery elm bark to form a poultice. Let it be applied cold, and changed three or four times a day, according to the degree of inflammation, until the swelling subsides or suppurates. When it is in an ulcerous state, it should be cleansed thoroughly with soap suds, and then washed or injected with a strong decoction of bayberry bark; then apply the following plaster: Take of bayberry tallow one part, white turpentine one part; melt, and add sweet oil, if necessary to soften it. Dress it in this manner once in twelve or twenty-four hours. The black or green salves may occasionally be substituted for the above salve, and changed. If there are deep sinuses, or holes, introduce the alkaline caustic, or a solution of it.

During the treatment of the tumor, or ulcer, the general alterative course should be pursued. Give the alterative powders, alterative syrup, and occasionally emetics, and the emetic and cathartic pills.

FEVER-SORES, OR ULCERS.

Fever-Sores present various appearances. Some are superficial sores, discharging simple purulent matter; others are deep-seated, and extend for considerable distance on the bone, with several openings, or holes, or with only one. In some cases, excrescences of fungus flesh form; others become callous, and hard about their edges; some are attended with violent inflammation, while others show but very little. These sores generally begin with swelling, and eventually ulcerate; sometimes small bruises degenerate into ulcers; they frequently follow violent attacks of fever, which falls into one limb, and from the use of mercury, which attacks some part, and causes swelling and ulceration.

TREATMENT.

The treatment of ulcers varies, according to their malignancy. The following indications naturally present themselves for consideration: To reduce inflammation, produce suppuration, cleanse the ulcer, remove fungus flesh, and induce a tendency to heal.

If the disease appears with violent swelling and inflammation, apply poultices to reduce it, and produce suppuration. For this purpose, apply the yest poultice, No. 43, alkaline, No. 44, or detergent, No. 47. When any part appears soft, and shows the presence of pus, or matter, an incision may be made, or a bit of the alkaline caustic applied, to cause an opening. When the sore begins to discharge, let it be thoroughly cleansed with soap suds, and syringed with vegetable elixir, or a tea of the detergent powders, No. 93, or bayberry bark, or with tincture of balsam of fir, and dressed with the green salve, with lobelia seed, pulverized; and repeat the syringing and dressing twice a day. If fungus flesh appear, or the margins of the sore appear dead or hard, apply the alkaline caustic.

In persons affected with these swellings, or ulcers, the constitution is always more or less affected, which may be the first exciting cause of them. It is therefore necessary to clear the system of these morbid affections. For this purpose, the general alterative course must be adopted: The alterative syrup and powders, the emetic and cathartic pills, and the vapor bath and emetics, should be attended to, according to the situation of the patient.

SCURVY SORES.

These are a species of fever-sores, and are called scurvy sores for distinction. They generally attack the legs. Their general appearance, is, a great swelling of the part, with a very high state of inflammation, attended with an intolerable sensation of burning and itching.—The skin becomes rough, or scaly; small pimples arise, which degenerate into small ulcers, with hard edges, or margins; the skin is sometimes livid, sometimes purple, at others nearly black.

TREATMENT.

The general course of treatment for this, is the same as for others, viz: Reduce the inflammation, heal the ulcers, and remove the irritation from the system. For removing the inflammation, apply the poultices—wash as directed for ulcers—dress with salve. The mineral water, No. 86, forms a wash of great value in this kind of sores, and an injection for ulcers. Steaming the parts with the infusion of bitter herbs, or water, is attended with decided advantage, and may be attended to at every dressing.

PILES.

Symptoms.—The first symptoms, are an uneasiness about the anus on going to stool, with a small protrusion of the rectum, with small hard tumors, which are often attended with discharges of blood, accompanying the stools, and occasionally at other times—with pain, burning, and itching of the parts.

TREATMENT.

The piles are simply a state of canker and inflammation of the lower intestines. The treatment, then, most proper, is such means as have a tendency to obviate these affections. For this purpose, give injections; the stimulating and emmolient may be used alternately, or a decoction of spikenard, comfrey, and bayberry, may also be used with warm medicine.

BLIND PILES.

This is a disease similar to the preceeding, in its causes and effects. The symptoms are, a sense of weight and uneasiness in the rectum, or lower intestines—sometimes with a sensation of pulsation, or beating, and heat; great pain in voiding the stools, attended with a distressing, death-like sensation, as it is often expressed; with weakness of the baek, and pain. This disease is sometimes mistaken for affections of the spine, in consequence of the effect it produces on that part.

TREATMENT.

The treatment for this species of piles, is the same as for the other species: The cold infusion of the pith of sassafras, drank for sometime, with the use of the warming medicine, will generally cure. The slippery elm bark is also a valuable article in this disease, taken in infusion, or added to the injections. When the piles are external, the apthalmic ointment is an excellent application.

Salt Rheum, Tetter.—*(Herpes.)*

This is a troublesome, inveterate eruption, appearing on different parts of the body, usually the hands. The appearances of this disease are various. Sometimes small vesicles, or eruptions, appear, which break and discharge a thin, ichorous, or corrosive matter, that causes extreme itching and irritation. After a while a scab forms, which, when rubbed off, will reappear.

It is attended with inflammation and swelling, and such a degree of itching and burning attend, that the patient is scarcely able to keep his hands from the parts affected. The parts sometimes become excoriated, stiff, and almost immoveable. It appears to be located principally underneath the skin, but the immediate cause is undoubtedly in the vascular system, or blood.

Other species, or other forms of the same disease, appear in the form of pustules, or blotches, which are at first distinct, and then spread together. Others appear on various parts of the body, in pimples and blotches.—Sometimes they appear in small, painful ulcers, which are in spots; these frequently spread, and produce large, foul ulcers, with considerable inflammation.

TREATMENT.

If the inflammation is considerable, apply poultices to reduce it; then apply the tetter ointment, or green salve, and wash with the mineral water; the tincture, in whiskey, of garden celendine, forms a valuable wash for these eruptions; but as the disease is in the blood, measures should be taken to remove it. For this purpose, a general alterative course should be pursued—as emetics, alterative powders, syrup, &c.

St. Anthony's Fire.—*(Erysipelas.)*

Erysipelas is a cutaneous inflammation, attended with redness, which disappears, and leaves a white spot for a short time after pressure with the finger, and shows a tendency to spread; the skin is a light rosy tint in the early stage. The cellular texture becomes affected, and a soft swelling of the part appears, which frequently involves a whole limb, and sometimes a considerable portion of the body. It sometimes attacks the face, at others the extremities, and most commonly the legs and ankles. The swelling is attended with high inflammation, throbbing, and peculiar pain. There is generally more or less constitutional disturbance, such as loss of appetite, head ache, nausea, febrile symptoms, disordered state of the stomach, weakness, dejection, &c.— The nearer the seat of the disease is to the head, the more violent these symptoms appear; and they sometimes extend to inflammation of the head, drowsiness, and delirium.

TREATMENT.

The object, in this disease, is to allay the inflammation, and attend to urgent symptoms. Where the symptoms are local only, the lobelia bitter fomentations, and the tincture of celendine, may be applied. Bandaging the parts will also have a tendency to reduce the inflammation and swelling. It is of the utmost importance to promote a general perspiration, and pursue the alterative course.

POISONS.

Poisons from ivy, sumach, and other vegetable poisons, generally produce great swelling, inflammation, and pain, which frequently proceed to ulceration, and become very foul and putrid.

TREATMENT.

Apply poultices to allay the inflammation. For this purpose, the detergent poultice is generally most suitable; then apply the elder ointment, or green salve, and wash the sores with soap suds, the tincture of lobelia, and a decoction of the detergent powders.

INDEX.

CPSIA information can be obtained at www.ICGtesting.com
228267LV00001B/7/A

9 781557 095831